# Beat Psoriasis

## The natural way

**Sandra Gibbons**

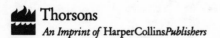

Thorsons
*An Imprint of* HarperCollins*Publishers*

Thorsons
An Imprint of HarperCollins*Publishers*
77–85 Fulham Palace Road,
Hammersmith, London W6 8JB
1160 Battery Street
San Francisco, California 94111-1213

Published by Thorsons 1992
10  9  8  7  6  5  4

A catalogue record for this book
is available from the British Library

ISBN 0 7225 2586 9

Printed in Great Britain by
Mackays of Chatham, Kent

A percentage of the royalties from this book will be
donated by the author to the Cancer First Aid Charity
that provides financial support within 48 hours to
cancer sufferers and their families.

# Beat Psoriasis

This book is dedicated to the memory of my father.

# Acknowledgements

I would like to thank all those wonderful people who so generously contributed valuable information, emotional support and encouragement, and practical help whilst I was writing this book.

In particular, special thanks to many of our patients and the staff at The Alternative Centre in London, and to Jane Waters and Toni Simmons, and the medical team, and patients from many countries, at the Dead Sea resort in Israel, and Israel Tsir-Cohen and Shmuel Zurel from the Israel Ministry of Tourism, for their practical assistance which was of great help.

Further, I would like to thank Kenneth Wingrove-Gibbons and Ruth Delman, founders of the Chi Traditional Chinese Medical Clinic who specialise in the treatment of eczema, Daniel Cromer, Sylvia Adler, Beverley Berg, Peter Todd, Hawkin Lovell, Peter McDonald, John Hardaker, Jane Judd, my literary agent, for her faith, and finally to Nicky Thomas for her help in completing the final draft.

# Contents

# Foreword

Psoriasis is a common skin condition, yet the understanding of its causes remains incomplete. Its traditional treatment has been of limited benefit, and so it is encouraging to sufferers and professionals to be addressed so directly in this book which explains a holistic approach to treating it.

There is much positive guidance and advice on lifestyle changes that not only treat psoriasis, but also maintain a healthy skin. The approach is completely natural and non-drug, emphasising at all times the involvement of the sufferer in his or her own treatment.

The Alternative Centre dedicates its work to the serious care of psoriasis sufferers, and this book is an excellent explanation of its aims and successes.

Dr Susan M. Horsewood-Lee
MB, BS, MRCGP
London

# Note to Reader

# Introduction

In the spring of 1986, a few months after the publication of my book, *Living with Psoriasis*, something miraculous happened. After 25 years as a sufferer, my psoriasis cleared and has remained clear to this date.

So, what is the secret that brought this about? It is the holistic approach – the only real way to relieve psoriasis. The holistic philosophy consists of learning to solve the physical, practical and psychological aspects of being a sufferer. It takes a little more time and effort, but I can assure you that this approach to the problem proved for me to be an effective therapy and a worthwhile investment in a new way of life – for the rest of my life. I have also personally seen the way this unique strategy has changed the lives of others, proving to be a virtual 'life saver' to many.

Since my recovery I have been teaching the holistic approach to relieving psoriasis to doctors, dermatologists, health care professionals and psoriasis sufferers internationally. In this book I will share with you my own and other successes I have experienced over the past ten years in my profession as an author, lecturer and specialist in holistic health education with many years experience in the field of psoriasis. I will continue to teach others around the world the holistic way to restore health. It worked for me, and it can work for you.

My story begins when, at the age of 14, psoriasis appeared on my face causing great distress and embarrassment. Disguising my condition and avoiding all activities involving the risk of discovery immediately became a way of life. I clearly remember the feelings of anxiety, lack of confidence, rejection and isolation along with many moments of fear of others finding out my 'secret'. Frequent visits to the family doctor offered no hope, just another prescription for the latest cream.

Eight years later, further lesions appeared, and still the most frequent advice given was: 'You will have to learn to live with it.' But no-one could suggest how. The power of the skin's appearance to attract or repel has been with us since the beginning of time, so a great deal of courage is needed to face the world when, in the words of many sufferers, 'you feel like a leper'.

Psoriasis is not only a condition of the skin but a many sided problem, causing medical, social, economic, sexual and emotional distress. A few years ago a lecturer in Sociology at St John's College, Cambridge, conducted a survey with psoriasis sufferers. He asked: 'What is the worst thing about having psoriasis?' 84 per cent said difficulties in establishing relationships and social contacts was the most distressing factor. Embarrassment and self-consciousness were also mentioned, as was the necessity to wear clothing that concealed their psoriasis.

A long time passed before I realised that much of the stigma I felt was in my imagination. What one person feels as a stigma, another does not. It can be used for all the misfortune that comes our way. I was guilty of associating my own prejudice with others. I felt badly about myself, so assumed others felt badly about me.

Occasionally I met someone insensitive, and I learnt to smile and say that I was not in this world to live up to their expectations. When asked what was wrong with my skin, I explained very clearly, taking care to emphasise that it was not catching.

Confidence and courage were what I needed if my life were to cease being a battle. I stopped searching for the 'promised cure', convinced that the answer to my dilemma lay within. Suddenly I began to feel a powerful sense of freedom. I had become a prisoner in my mind, making my own laws. I should have felt grateful I was not suffering from a more serious handicap or life-threatening disease.

It was not my psoriasis causing feelings of loneliness and rejection, it was the way I was coping with it. Why should I feel ashamed? I had done nothing wrong, I just had psoriasis. Now was the time to step out of the darkness into the light, allowing my mind to become the healer not the slayer. The next step was to investigate the claim that diet could help psoriasis.

A prominent naturopathic practitioner volunteered for this role. He recommended a regime of salads, fruit and mineral water, with the inclusion of dried apricots and almonds. After ten weeks my psoriasis cleared for the first time in 18 years.

It proved to be a simple case of raw foods eliminating the toxins from the body, as with the process of fasting. (None of these diets should be undertaken without professional advice.) My belief that the answer to psoriasis lay in the total health of the mind and body strengthened by the day.

The next task was to re-adjust the diet to suit my personal needs and lifestyle – and remain clear of psoriasis. I succeeded six years later just by eliminating dairy foods from my normal, less restrictive diet. It was that simple.

During those six years, along with two colleagues, Jane Waters, a fellow sufferer, and Toni Simmons, whose daughters were afflicted, we decided to open the Alternative Centre in London. The aim of the centre, the only one of its kind in the world, was to teach others like ourselves how to cope more easily with the problems psoriasis presents in our daily lives. It was an uphill struggle to gain recognition, but we persevered with the knowledge that there were millions of you all over the world, needing practical help and advice on how to achieve the quality of life you deserved.

After nearly ten years of specialising in psoriasis, our work at the Centre has become internationally recognised for its valuable contribution towards the health of others. Over 10,000 sufferers have found their way to us, many of whom have contributed towards the research for this book. Other contributions have come from research carried out at the Alternative Centre and the International Psoriasis Solarium at the Dead Sea resort in Israel, world famous for its truly unique healing environment, that without doubt has also proved to be a 'life saver' to psoriasis sufferers from all over the world for many years.

Further contributions also come from my attendance at international seminars, meeting delegates from the conventional and natural medicine fields, and from my lectures at overseas dermatology conferences. I have also consulted with trainee dermatologists at Radcliffe Hospital in Oxford, met with European psoriasis associations, participated in psoriasis phone-ins with BBC radio, made television appearances, and conducted interviews with the media.

Support, encouragement and requests to write this book have come from all over the world, for which I am eternally thankful. My new way of life offers me the opportunity to spend the rest of my life teaching others how they, too, can gain the quality of life they deserve.

# Chapter 1

# The holistic approach

A consultation at the Alternative Centre usually takes around two hours, and during this time patients are taught the holistic approach to healing their psoriasis. At the initial consultation, notes are taken on a patient's general medical history – what treatments they have received in the past for any illness that may have occurred – and then their history and treatment of psoriasis is discussed in depth. At this point they are encouraged to express their feelings about suffering from this condition and the problems it has created at whatever level. It is often the first time they have spoken to someone who understands how they feel. At the Centre we have all had experience of being psoriasis sufferers.

Patients are made aware of dietary advice, lifestyle counselling and the way stress factors influence our lives and the effect they can have on the physical organs of our body, of which the skin is a reflection. In our experience it is vital that the patient understands what holistic medicine is, as they have to be willing to play their part in the healing process. Disease means 'disharmony' and, since the mind influences the body, distress, suppressed emotions, feelings of rejection, loneliness and many other negative thought patterns can have a devastating effect on our total health. These create an imbalance which results in disharmony. Psoriasis conditions can fluctuate dramatically, with varying percentages of lesions occurring at different times. They wax and wane, or perhaps go into remission – all this is a reflection of the emotional, psychological and physical state of a sufferer's health.

A negative reaction to stress over a period of time can take its toll on our systems of digestion and elimination, resulting in a build-up of toxins, and in the body's desperate attempt to stay healthy, the skin, another major elimination organ, overflows with toxins as it starts to become an alternative disposal system. So when you apply an external cream or treatment to the psoriasis when the body is trying to release the toxins via the skin it is a bit like putting a lid on a pot that is boiling over.

## Mora-Therapy Unit

To monitor a patient's condition a Mora-Therapy unit is used. These units are widely used by medical professionals in Europe for the purpose of diagnosing the degeneration of the physical organs of the body – so that, for instance, the onset of kidney disease could be recognised and treated before a patient actually started experiencing the symptoms. Its role in preventative medicine is becoming increasingly renowned. This small, efficient unit registers the electro-magnetic field of each organ of the body via the energy pathways – known as meridians in the practice of the 5000 year-old therapy of acupuncture. A probe is placed on the terminal acupuncture points on the hands and feet which correspond to the organs being tested. The test is simple to apply and there is no discomfort. No needles are used in this procedure. An electro-magnetic reading is taken of the patient's lymphatic system, lungs, large intestine, nervous system, circulation system, backache-degeneration, digestive system, heart, small intestine, spleen, pancreas, liver, joints, stomach, connective tissues (muscles and ligaments), skin, fatty tissue, gall bladder, kidneys and bladder. Patients are able to see for themselves any internal energy imbalance. This is a vital lesson in learning how their general health affects the condition of their psoriasis. The dial on the Mora-Therapy unit reads from 0-100 and a patient's reading would be 50 in every energy field if their body were in perfect working order.

At this stage in their holistic programme patients usually begin to show genuine excitement about the journey they are to begin on their road to recovery. We feel this breakthrough occurs when they realise that they control their own level of health. All we have to do is show them the way. As Jane Waters says to each patient during their consultation with her: 'We can give you all the information you need to heal yourself. What you decide to do with that information is your decision. We will show you how to trigger your own self-healing process, the rest is up to you.' But for most it is the first time they have experienced a sense of joy and hope. What many find frightening at first is the sense of responsibility they have to have for themselves if they want to achieve any measure of success.

The diagram shows a patient's reading from the Mora-Therapy unit, and it can be seen that all the energy systems of this particular patient are out of balance. This is not uncommon. The next step is to identify which energy system is the cause behind this total imbalance which is affecting the patient's skin. Common amongst causes are wrong eating habits, addictions, chemical and environmental pollution, excess alcohol, caffeine, previous illnesses, after-effects of medications, immunisations, extensive dental work, hereditary factors, injuries and psychological and emotional disturbances.

Out of the 126 cases of psoriasis treated, 115 showed an imbalance in the lungs, 126 the colon, 124 the digestive system, 125 the liver, and 125 the kidneys.

Careful analysis of the readings from the Mora-Therapy unit and information gained from the patient in consultation leads to a careful selection process of remedies from natural sources, high in vibrational energy, that are complementary to the patient's self-healing process. Remedies that will assist in restoring and rejuvenating the patient's own healing energy. They also help in releasing accumulative excess toxins. Detoxifying the physical body is the key to healing the skin and releasing your own healing energy.

This form of alternative therapy also has a remarkable effect on some of the psychological and emotional disturbances so common with psoriasis sufferers. Once they see their skin beginning to improve many of their negative thought processes automatically disappear without psychotherapy. Each patient's needs on both physical and psychological levels are unique. Some will respond well to homoeopathically-prepared remedies, others to extracts from the healing properties of certain plants, and often a combination is recommended.

The next series of tests relate directly to the skin. Products are tested for their compatibility to the patient's skin – to ensure the best possible chance of the patient's maximum benefit with the minimum amount of distress. From the

## Mora-Therapy Test Reading

**Patient's Name:**  **Date:**  **Right**  **Left**

| Point chosen | | 1 | 2 | |
|---|---|---|---|---|
| Hand | LY | 42 | 50 | |
| | LU | 47 | 50 | |
| | CO | 42 | 50 | |
| | NS | 43 | 50 | |
| | CS | 39 | 50 | |
| | AL | 42 | 50 | |
| | DEG | 45 | 50 | |
| | TW | 42 | 50 | |
| | HT | 47 | 50 | |
| | SI | 47 | 50 | |

| Point chosen | | 1 | 2 | |
|---|---|---|---|---|
| Foot | SP | 47 | 50 | |
| | LI | 41 | 50 | |
| | JT | 41 | 50 | |
| | ST | 52 | 50 | |
| | CT | 42 | 50 | |
| | SK | 42 | 50 | |
| | FT | 55 | 50 | |
| | GBL | 48 | 50 | |
| | KI | 48 | 50 | |
| | BL | 39 | 50 | |

enormous selection of treatments available for psoriasis sufferers to apply to the skin we only choose those to recommend that are natural, safe, easy-to-apply and pleasant to use. After many years of suffering and dealing with psoriasis ourselves we are well and truly experienced in knowing what psoriasis sufferers *do not want*.

The product ranges include bath solutions, soaps and shampoos, and treatments for the irritation, redness, flaking, soreness and extreme dryness. We also recommend that any other substances that come into contact with the skin be tested for compatibility with a patient's skin. These may be shaving preparations, cosmetics, hair treatments, toiletries, washing powders or chemicals.

## *Diet*

Advice is given on dietary adjustments and how an excess of certain foods can have a harmful effect on the organs of the body. This also applies to food additives. Also covered are preparation procedures and what utensils are used. Cooking methods are discussed – microwave ovens and your health, aluminium cooking pans – as are nutrient and energy requirements.

## Environmental factors

The next question that arises concerns the home environment and how improvements can be made to reduce the bad effects of anything that might aggravate your psoriasis – central heating, for example, can increase irritation. Recommendations are made for alternative products for cleaning, and how to prevent cuts and abrasions. All the physical, practical and psychological ways you can overcome these problems that affect those with psoriasis are covered in the rest of this book.

Another area is that of electro-magnetic pollution and geopathic stress. Although a controversial subject there is growing evidence that such stresses can adversely affect our health. If you understand that our bodies consist of an electro-magnetic field then it makes sense that any added electrical influences may have the potential to imbalance our systems. In the last few decades we have been increasingly bombarded by many forms of electro-magnetic radiation from modern communications technology.

Scientists have also been looking at the subject of geopathic stress and how it affects our health. Many disorders have been associated with this phenomenon, like cancer, multiple sclerosis, impotence, infertility, allergies, skin rashes, cysts and many more. Geopathic stress is associated with the natural rays which rise up from the earth's mantle. It is said to be caused by the distortion of the mantle by weak electro-magnetic fields created by underground cavities, mineral concentrations, and subterranean water courses. When there is resistance to treatment, it could be due to a patient being subjected to geopathic stress.

Patients living in the country are often in despair during the crop spraying season because of the inflamed condition of their skin. Chemicals from the dry cleaning of clothes, and dyes used in fabrics, can be a problem for psoriasis sufferers, and it is often found that patients are suffering from the chemicals they come into contact with at their work. A double glazing salesman, for example, was affected by the cutting and manufacturing processes at the factory he visited for his stock. As he was only in this vicinity for a couple of hours each week it did not occur to him to wear protective clothing. Sufferers who move to urban areas also quite frequently experience a worsening of their psoriasis.

Every occupation has its hazards, and such day-to-day stresses need to be taken into account during the consultation process when sufferers seek help. It is then mutually decided what other forms of treatment or complementary therapy might accelerate a patient's healing process. At times a programme is recommended which may incorporate relaxation therapy, meditation, deep breathing, stress therapy and even psychotherapy. Sometimes patients are referred to a specialist medical doctor for a blood test or other relevant health checks. Above all a sympathetic listener seems to be the most popular need.

## *Speed of recovery*

The time it takes for an improvement in a patient's psoriasis condition and in their general health varies according to the length of the programme, but on average a change is seen within 12 weeks. It must be realized, though, that as many sufferers have had their psoriasis for 10-20-30 years they cannot expect to experience dramatic improvements in the first part of their holistic healing programme. The body heals from the inside out so the skin tends to heal last. The holistic programme has nevertheless proved a more long lasting and successful way of treating psoriasis than simply treating the symptom with skin applications.

The second part of the programme is usually when a more dramatic improvement will be noticed on the skin. Many patients clear their psoriasis completely, and then learn preventative measures that they can apply themselves to enable them to control their health and avoid a return of their psoriasis. It is this new-found experience of feeling in control that has proved to be so effective in the holistic approach to healing psoriasis.

# Case histories

There follow some case histories to help you to truly understand what the holistic programme involves.

One case is of a young man who had spent most of his life in agricultural work overseas in third world countries. Due to the nature of his job he had been subjected to many immunisations. He had also been treated many times with antibiotics since the age of nine and had twice been a victim of tropical diseases. His psoriasis had begun 15 years previously after an accident in which he received burns. He was at the time treated with tranquillizers, morphine, and penicillin. So, you can see, he had received more than his fair share of drug-related treatments.

The result of his Mora-Therapy test was that large and small intestine, digestive system, stomach and liver were showing severe signs of stress. In addition to his recommended de-toxification programme he was given a traditional homoeopathic remedy to help correct these disorders. Adjustments to his diet were also recommended.

After six weeks there was already a remarkable improvement in his psoriasis. He had cleared it by 50%, the remaining lesions having faded in colour considerably, and his discomfort had been relieved.

Particular attention was paid in the course of his treatment to de-toxifying his liver and to easing his digestive process. The long history of medication and immunisation had weakened his internal organs and immune system, so it was important to restore the balance in his body. The improvement he experienced encouraged him to continue the holistic healing programme for a further four months in order to maximise his chances of long-term relief. He was advised how to overcome a possible reoccurence of his psoriasis, due to any further immunisation or medication. Effective homoeopathic treatments can eliminate some of the reactions and prevent the skin becoming worse or new lesions breaking out. Other factors which were discussed included how to avoid food poisoning, dietary precautions and hygiene practice to minimise the risk of infections. He now only has a few spots of psoriasis remaining, and is presently overseas on a two-year assignment.

Another case history involves a lady of 35 who had become a sufferer at the age of 13. She had a long history of steroid treatments, methotrexate and coal tar applications. Her limbs, face and scalp were affected, often accompanied by a burning sensation.

She had heard of Pharbifarm, a natural skin formula, and had been using it for about one year with improvement. She decided to visit the Centre for further help, and it was found that she also suffered from female problems and there were some emotional influences in her life that were affecting her health, as well as her psoriasis. Her liver showed obvious signs of overstress, and most of her other organs were out of balance. She was put on a de-toxifying programme, and she continued this at home in her own country.

One of the motivating factors in wanting to heal herself was a growing wish to help fellow psoriasis sufferers in her country. It was as though she had discovered a new lease of life and after three months treatment her psoriasis was clear. So, she achieved her dream, in that she is now an inspiration to others and, having learnt all she could to help others with psoriasis, she has started her own self-help therapy service where she teaches other sufferers how they can heal their skin.

A patient in his mid-fifties, a businessman and grandfather, was found to be a very keen drinker of tea (20-30 cups a day). He showed a great deal of reluctance at the thought of having to moderate this habit, as he had never before considered this to have been a contributory factor towards the worsening of his psoriasis or that it was damaging his health.

As with many patients, he could not perceive it could be so simple to heal his skin. He had been a sufferer for over 15 years with a 25% coverage, but for most of this time he tried to ignore it except for the occasional visit to his doctor for creams. One day he woke up and decided he had to find a permanent solution to his psoriasis. The contributory factor to this decision, as occurs with so many sufferers, was that he had decided for the first time in years to take a holiday and was eager to improve his condition before his exposure to the sun.

He was advised to slowly cut down his tea drinking, and to make adjustments to his diet as part of a de-toxifying process. This included the avoidance of processed foods and tap water. After six weeks his psoriasis had cleared by 50%. Reducing his tea drinking to just two cups a day had certainly been worthwhile. Needless to say, he enjoyed his holiday and has not returned to his previous tea drinking habit.

Another case is of a 35 year old lady who was happily married with two young children. She had been a sufferer since her father died when she was a teenager. Her mother suffers with severe arthritis, and the case involved the mother and daughter being treated together because of the family's emotional and business problems.

Her psoriasis lesions were on her scalp, arms, legs, and front and back of her body – about a 40% coverage which caused her great distress as her work brought her in touch with the public every day. She had previously taken the normal medical route as well as attempting all types of natural remedies, like cod liver oil, evening primrose oil and different combinations of vitamins and minerals and cosmetic creams. Anything anyone told her would work she spent her money on to no avail.

The Mora-Therapy showed symptoms of digestive disturbances, and every energy system was out of balance. A gentle de-toxification process was recommended, as it was apparent these toxins had accumulated over many years. In addition to the more common toxins, her body had been severely overloaded by excessive self-administered supplements, placing extra stress on her liver. Her diet needed only minimal adjustment, but she was advised to stop using tap water. After being given her personal holistic programme, which included applications for the skin and advice on precautionary measures, she was advised to return after six weeks for a review.

On the second visit a visible difference was seen in her psoriasis in that flaking, irritations and soreness was diminished and the redness had begun to pale. The next step was to continue the de-toxification programme for a further four weeks and during this time her skin showed even more improvement, including the disappearance of some of her lesions.

She was unable to return for a further visit for two months because of very stressful family and business commitments. Even so, during this time, she succeeded in keeping her psoriasis in its newly improved condition. However, there were no signs of further improvement. Another visit was encouraged, and it was suggested she be accompanied by her mother who, it was known, had a great deal of influence on her daughter's life. It was now necessary to find the reason for the healing block that had occurred, and emotional and psychological disturbances were revealed during a two hour consultation with the psoriasis sufferer, and an hour with the mother. This helped them both a great deal as they managed to solve many differences they had been afraid to admit to before.

A few adjustments were made to the remedies for the patient, and the mother visited a few weeks later when further counselling was given. Eight weeks after that, the daughter reported her psoriasis totally cleared, and she remained clear thereafter.

A very houseproud housewife in her late 50s, visited the Centre for help for her hands which were swollen, blistered and cracked, and extremely painful. Her feet were also in a bad condition. Her condition had waxed and waned for many years, and she had tried all manner of medical treatments from her doctor, and as a hospital out-patient. The year before her visit had been an extremely distressing one for her, and her condition had become chronic. Difficult as it may be to understand, it was actually because she was unable to carry out her household chores with her usual high degree of perfection because of the condition of her hands. It was discovered that her hands had suddenly become more worse after her husband had retired.

On her first visit her hands and feet were so swollen it was not possible to get any accurate readings on the Mora-Therapy unit. Most of the consulting time was spent advising on all the precautions she had to take to protect her hands and feet. For example the rubber gloves she was having to use during washing up made her hands worse. A great deal of counselling was necessary to deal with her obsessional behaviour concerning her house cleaning, and with her frustration at not being able to use her hands to carry this out.

Flower essences, known for helping patients showing psychological disturbances, were recommended and she was put on the holistic de-toxification programme. One of the most important objectives for this patient was for her to find another interest in her life. Not only was she adjusting to her husband's retirement but she felt he was in the way of her cleaning. The condition of her psoriasis was very clearly linked with these factors, and a liver disorder was also revealed on her second check-up.

Her liver had been affected by PUVA treatment and other medications she had taken for her skin. De-toxification of her liver was where therapy was mainly focused. Creams were recommended for helping to stop soreness.

Both she and her husband had reached a time in their lives when they felt it was over and they had nothing left to look forward to. All the possible alternative interests to housework she wanted to pursue involved her hands. She was therefore encouraged to think about and prepare herself for starting her newly chosen interests once her hands had healed. She needed to feel she had a purpose in life.

A few weeks later the swelling on her hands had gone down, as a result of the de-toxification programme that was helping to restore her liver and improve her energy levels. Her treatment continued for a couple of months subsequently, and during this time she started evening classes to study needlework and knitting, showing particular interest in design – something she had never envisaged before her therapy. She now teaches those subjects at the school. About six months after her first consultation her hands and feet were clear of psoriasis, and she was able to live a happier life.

## The will to get better

It is not claimed that sufferers are 'cured', and certainly not all of them clear their condition. Apart from the treatments they follow, the important thing is what changes they are prepared to make in their lives to overcome their problem. Many sufferers, even with severe psoriasis, do not actually want to get well, or simply don't have the energy to try. In Israel I discovered that some sufferers, visiting the Dead Sea to clear their condition, felt that if they stayed clear after returning home for too long they would not feel justified – or perhaps their partners would not allow them – to take such a break each year away from all the stresses of every-day life.

I feel that by teaching you our unique natural, healthy way of living – a holistic programme of self-help techniques carefully chosen to enable you to achieve optimum health, that can be integrated into your daily life, with the minimum of fuss and inconvenience – your psoriasis can clear and stay clear.

At the Centre, our future plans are to teach sufferers who clear their skin, and who want to start a new career, to become Holistic Practitioners in order that they too may be an inspiration to others, showing them how to restore their health.

# Chapter 2

# Choosing the right treatment

I have heard many stories, some amusing, some distressing of fortunes being spent on searching for the 'right treatment'. One lady from Austria, was advised by a dentist she consulted, whilst living in Germany, to have her teeth removed, at great expense. 'This is the right treatment for you, it will cure your psoriasis', she was told. The lady decided that after many years of suffering it was worth a try. She still has her psoriasis today and no teeth of her own. A well known psychotherapist told of a patient who had been advised to go to India to see a specialist, who had the 'right treatment' for him. He returned to London, after taking a dubious herbal mixture and was rushed into hospital seriously ill. Thankfully, he has since fully recovered.

A 'cure', costing £1,000 for some tablets, came to my attention some years ago. The terms of the treatment were that the money would have to be paid in advance, but would be refunded if the 'cure' was unsuccessful. The source moved to different parts of the country at regular intervals, perhaps to avoid the promised refunds. Details of a complicated diet were offered for sale from a business address in the North of England. Follow this diet and you will be 'cured' was the claim. You were sworn to absolute secrecy as to the content of the diet, obviously in an attempt to secure further sales to psoriasis sufferers. The diet had no effect on the patient. The sum of £30,000 was spent, travelling the world, by a young man from Nigeria in a quest to find *his* 'cure', but to no avail.

Many of you will already be aware of the burden placed on you and your family in getting treatment for what seems to be an incurable condition. We all agree that if the flaking and irritation could be alleviated, we could cope with the rest of the disabling effects of psoriasis. As you know, some treatments offered seem worse than having the condition itself. They so often smell unpleasant and are difficult and messy to use, staining your skin, clothes, bed linen and other household fabrics. In one sad case, a sufferer was asked to leave his family home as his mother could no longer tolerate the tar products her son had to use.

We have all had experience of marginally effective treatments which are often impractical and unpleasant to use. These are prescribed by some doctors, many of whom underestimate how psoriasis affects the lives of their patients. More and more psoriasis sufferers are now tending to turn to alternative and complementary medicine as they become aware of the side-effects of long-term drug treatments.

The following information will help you choose the right treatment:

## *Ultraviolet light*

Reports are that the positive effects of UVB are changing the lives of psoriasis sufferers everywhere. Pioneered in Sweden by Professor Gunnar Swanbeck, one of the world's leading professors of dermatology and an internationally recognised authority on the subject and treatment of psoriasis – ultraviolet light therapy has been studied and used in hospitals for over 20 years in Sweden. It certainly seems to be the least of all evils, particularly in relation to severe psoriasis, and with the availability of home-use UVB units it has become a therapy which can be used with minimal disruption of normal life.

It is increasingly popular in Scandinavia and other European countries, since it meets patients' needs for a more convenient treatment, and has become the most common psoriasis therapy in many medical centres.

It is well known that summer is the best season for most psoriasis sufferers. Sunshine is a good medicine and the skin can improve considerably, with symptoms often disappearing completely. Hence the development of the use of 'artificial sunlight' in the form of ultraviolet light treatment. Today it is known that it is the UVB rays that are most effective against psoriasis.

The sun's rays comprise an electromagnetic spectrum. The spectrum includes radio waves, microwaves, infra-red radiation (heat), X-rays, gamma rays, visible and ultraviolet. They are measured and classified in the spectrum according to the wavelength. Ultraviolet spans the wavelength between 400-100 nanometres (a nanometre is one thousand millionth of a metre and is abbreviated to read nm). It is further subdivided into three types of ultraviolet rays, expressed as UVA (400-315nm), UVB (315-280nm) and UVC (280-100nm).

UVA rays are closest to the visible spectrum. They pass through ordinary window glass and are known for their cosmetic effect in darkening the pigment of the skin. UVA itself has little effect on psoriasis. UVB cannot pass through ordinary window glass, but it is this part of the spectrum that produces all of the biological effects following exposure to sunlight. It is here we find the positive effects on psoriasis. UVC rays do not concern us in the treatment of psoriasis as this wavelength does not normally pass through the earth's atmosphere, but the hole in the ozone layer is now allowing harmful UVC rays to penetrate the earth's atmosphere, and is becoming a matter of increasing concern.

## Is selective UVB necessary?

Studies have been carried out to find the exact UVB wavelengths that produce the maximum clearance of psoriasis with the minimum risk. Results suggest that eliminating wavelengths less than 296nm may improve the effect. Using a so-called 'monochromatic' UVB source at 300nm, 304nm and 313nm psoriasis that had quickly returned to sites previously exposed to 'broadband' UVB cleared. Additionally broadband UVA (320nm-400nm) seen to be effective in clearing psoriasis from small exposure sites, showed UVB to be as effective in doses 1,000 times less.

Selective UVB rays, known as selective ultraviolet phototherapy (SUP), are now manufactured in line with these findings, emitting a continuous spectrum of 270-400nm with a peak at 313nm. It is interesting to note that the standard spectrum emitted from a UVA solarium (traditionally for suntanning) is between 305-445nm with a peak at 350nm.

## UVB in use

Many dermatology units in hospitals and clinics throughout the world now use UVB for the treatment of psoriasis. Indeed in Scandinavian countries the use of ultraviolet light therapy is almost a tradition, and now more than 20 years of good experience has led them to pioneer day care centres. With no appointments necessary, and open in the evenings as well as during the day, patients can visit for treatment on their way to and from work enabling them to lead as normal a life as possible. A few hospitals in the UK are now endeavouring to expand on this idea.

Now, too, home solarium treatment of psoriasis is available. Provided the patient is fully trained in its correct and controlled use, the lucky ones who react positively to the sun (and fortunately this is by far the majority) can now benefit all the year round in their own homes. But the easy purchase of UVB units for home use is the cause of some concern to doctors and dermatologists, and certain criteria must be met in order to balance the risk/benefit ratios.

- The unit must satisfy high standards of reliability, function and safety.
- Diagnosis must be confirmed by a doctor or dermatologist prior to use.
- Certain drugs produce phototoxic or photoallergic reactions. They are few in number but patients receiving treatment for any other condition or illness must be carefully screened.
- Long-term users of topical steroids (not unusual amongst psoriasis sufferers) must be assessed with extreme care.
- In the event of pregnancy a doctor's or dermatologist's advice should be sought.
- The patient needs to know whether or not they benefit from the sun.
- Counselling is required in order to assess the patient's correct skin type. There are now internationally accepted categories of skin types that help define this. The type of skin determines the correct exposure time required in order to receive the exact erythema dose (erythema is a slight redness that should occur within 24 hours after each treatment, if the exposure time is correct).
- Patients should be aware of the importance of carefully measuring the distance between themselves and the UVB light unit.
- Patients who are outdoor workers, or are otherwise exposed

to a lot of sunlight in daily life, should be advised to cover their face and hands and/or feet if they have no skin lesions in these areas.

● Goggles must be worn. Natural sun rays contain so much visible light that our reflexes make us look away. With any ultraviolet therapy the amount of visible light is so small that our reflexes do not function. Even nurses attending patients using ultraviolet light are advised to wear eye protection.

● Check-ups by a dermatologist are encouraged on a regular basis.

If these criteria are met, then UVB home solarium treatment can be of enormous benefit to thousands of psoriasis sufferers.

## Is UVB treatment for psoriasis safe?

Short term side-effects of burning and blistering with redness are uncomfortable but not dangerous and can be totally avoided if detailed instructions are followed with care.

Wrinkling of the skin (actinic elastosis) and skin malignancies are associated with long-term exposure to direct sunshine, and whether similar risk factors exist with the use of UVB units is under investigation. Studies in Sweden, with accurate records kept over more than 20 years, show no increase in actinic elastosis or skin malignances in a control population matched for sex, age and geographical residence. A typical psoriasis patient has to be on UVB treatment for 5-10 years to reach the average of treatments recorded in the study. Neither skin type nor sex seemed to be of significance. However, a pattern of advanced age and outdoor occupation did prove to be risk factors. A comparison was made between the amount of UVB received in psoriasis treatment and various outdoor vacational activities. The results indicate that the therapeutic doses are not appreciably higher than may be received by active sunbathing for the same period during the summer months in Sweden.

The inhabitants of Sweden get a relatively small amount of UVB from natural sunlight as with most northerly latitude countries, although this may change in time with the effects of global warming.

# To UVB or not to UVB

The effectiveness of UVB treatment is shown to be superior to that of topical steroids; similar to dithranol and coal tar but much more convenient to use, and its side-effects are generally considered milder than for PUVA or methotrexate.

There are a large number of studies showing the positive effect of UVB on psoriasis. Generally patients will be clear of lesions with five treatments per week. Good results are often obtained with only three treatments per week. The patient has to spend between 1½-15 minutes per treatment, and on average lesions are cleared within less than two months, leaving the skin free of symptoms for another two months, and having only mild symptoms for a further two months.

The risks involved with UVB are about the same as becoming an outdoor worker who is exposed to sunlight daily. When considering risk-benefit factors of UVB for treatment of psoriasis it must also be remembered that most other forms of medical psoriasis treatment have their risks too. We must also accept that some treatments suit some sufferers and not others.

To UVB or not to UVB is not a question of life or death. It may, however, be a question of the quality of life for the psoriasis sufferer.

In 1984 the leading professor of dermatology in Sweden requested that The Alternative Centre make available the Swedish government-approved Corona Climate Therapy Units to psoriasis sufferers in the UK for home use.

They have proved to a popular therapy allowing sufferers to clear their condition in the privacy of their own home, thus avoiding unnecessary hospitalization where severe cases are concerned. Once the patient has cleared, with practical after care education on how to stay clear using the holistic approach, they are able to minimize long-term usage of UVB.

Do not waste your money buying a UVA sunbed to clear your psoriasis. They are for tanning purposes only.

# Pharbifarm formulas

These were developed in Sweden nearly 20 years ago by a Swedish chemist who suffered from psoriasis, and they have become well known internationally for their effectiveness in helping psoriasis sufferers cope with the dryness and flaking of their skin. Such was the success of the Pharbifarm drug-free range of cosmetic treatments that they were the subject of debate in the Swedish parliament in March 1975.

The Pharbifarm range is a natural, safe alternative to the more toxic substances most commonly recommended for treatment of skin conditions.

*Formula 1* is a special blend of extract of herbs and mineral salts.

*Formula 2* is a unique combination of natural plant oils.

The shampoo, used in combination with formulas No. 1 and No. 2 for the scalp, is detergent-free and 100% soluble.

The *Bath Formula* is an effective lubricant that protects the skin from the harsh elements of the water, and the soap will lubricate the skin.

This range of skin care has been available for the past 20 years and has been recommended by doctors, dermatologists and health care professionals to many thousands of psoriasis sufferers. Many of whom will testify, like myself, that it is easy and pleasant to use, with no unpleasant side-effects associated with short-term or long-term use.

## Choosing an alternative practitioner

For a patient wanting to take advantage of the treatments offered by practitioners of alternative, or complementary, medicine it can be an enormous problem. How can you tell who is well-qualified and who is not? It is reported that many hundreds of alternative practitioners are trained each year. Diplomas may be available by post to anyone willing to pay, and it is possible for someone with no formal expert training, but merely knowledge gained from a week-end course or from books, to offer their services to the public.

Choosing the wrong practitioner can be expensive and distressing, especially for psoriasis sufferers, as many 'miracle cures' can be offered. There is a risk that, because of poor training, an incorrect diagnosis can be made. Care also needs to be taken that there is no conflict between alternative treatment and any conventional treatment being used. It is advisable for patients to tell their doctors if they are undergoing alternative therapy, and always be sure that your diagnosis is made by a medical professional.

Do not be afraid to ask your doctor to recommend a good, experienced practitioner to you. Many doctors today are familiar with the practice of alternative therapies, and some encourage their use. Failing this, ask around. Word of mouth is another good way to find the right practitioner. Alternatively, telephone an established natural health centre. They normally have this information to hand.

How do you know which therapy is the best one for your particular complaint? First, ask the professional you have consulted exactly what the treatment is that he or she is recommending; the cost, side-effects if any, and the success rate – remembering also to check the duration of the treatment. It is important that the therapist understands the condition of psoriasis. So many don't.

There are a growing number of therapies that can help some of the symptoms of psoriasis – homoeopathy, acupuncture, herbalism, osteopathy, psychotherapy, spiritual healing, naturopathy. Not so widely acknowledged are such therapies as colour therapy, crystal healing, reflexology, iridology, hair analysis, aromatherapy and many more.

The human body responds to many different treatment methods, and perhaps alternative practitioners and medical doctors will one day unite their skills more fully, and lead us towards a truly holistic approach to healing – the right treatment for us all.

Meanwhile, I have chosen for you what our years of research have shown to be the 'right treatment' for psoriasis sufferers.

## Health spas and clinics

There are, of course, health spas and clinics around the world offering a wide range of natural therapies that may be combined with a relaxing vacation. Mainly these centres are used for rebuilding good health, not just treating a disease. For thousands of years spas have contributed towards the prevention of disease and to the healing and improvement of chronic conditions.

European countries have a 2,000 year tradition of spa treatment. The Romans restored their battle-weary bodies in hot mineral springs. Spa therapy without doubt does help to regenerate and rejuvenate the body. The Soviet Union has 3,500 spas. All over the world there are thousands of people who take spa therapy as part of their daily life. In Europe there are strict laws governing national spas and the treatment used. In Russia there are research institutes where continuous research is carried out in order to maximise results.

Naturopathy is the basis of most spa therapies. Finding the real cause of the illness and eliminating it, so that the body can heal itself. The therapy will include sunshine, recreation, rest, pleasant surroundings, exercise, dietary guidance, massage, electrotherapy, hydrotherapy, fasting and counselling if necessary. Specific treatment for psoriasis is offered in some spas, using mineral waters, fasting, application of creams for the skin and relaxation. Doctors or dermatologists are usually in attendance, and in many cases these therapies have helped psoriasis sufferers.

These natural health spas can be found in many countries. In Tiberias – in Israel, possibly the oldest spa in the world, they have natural hot springs containing valuable minerals, known to be effective for skin treatment. In beautiful surroundings, near the Sea of Galilee, this historic place has given skin sufferers at least temporary improvement.

In Iceland there is a natural health centre offering relief from psoriasis which involves the use of natural spring waters and treatment from a dermatologist. So far, little is known of its effectiveness. Another such centre is in Leysin, in Switzerland. Set in the mountains, this clinic, famous for the treatment of diabetes many years ago, has now become known for the treatment of psoriasis. The therapy is based on UVB light, if necessary, dietary advice and fumaric acid therapy, that has to be continued after you return home. It makes an ideal summer or winter vacation, but the lasting effectiveness of the treatment is primarily dependent on the long-term use of fumaric acid.

In Turkey a rather bizarre treatment for psoriasis has emerged. It involves immersing yourself in water filled with many thousands of small fish who then proceed to eat all the scales from your skin. According to reports, the sensation is not very comfortable and the improvement very temporary.

In Austria, West Germany, Italy, France, Czechoslovakia, Bulgaria and Mexico, there are said to be health spas and treatment centres specialising in skin conditions. Reports claim that some improvement of psoriasis has been seen, but cases of total clearance seem to be rare.

A Health holiday – the pleasant, fun way to clear your skin, and one that can be shared by partners and family. It could be the right treatment for you.

The Institute of Santa Monica in Poland is a branch of The Holistic Hospital in Santa Monica in Mexico, one of the largest health care establishments in the world for alternative treatment. This holistic clinic offers advanced naturopathic care combined with a vacation, and has successfully treated rheumatism, candidiasis, dental galvanism, tumour diseases, multiple sclerosis and heart and vascular disorders. There is also a possibility that effective treatment for psoriasis will be included at the Institute in Poland for those unable to go to the Dead Sea. For further information about this, contact the Alternative Centre (details at the back of this book).

## Health treatment vacations – at the Dead Sea in Israel

As a Dead Sea specialist, I have met many hundreds of psoriasis and arthritis sufferers on my frequent visits to Israel over the past few years and have witnessed the healing affects and listened to many points of view from patients of all nationalities. This international place offers sanctuary to people who have never before experienced relief of their psoriasis in such a pleasant, healthy way with such long-lasting results.

There are four clinics for sufferers in the area, The Mor Dermatological and Rheumatological Clinic, The Ein Bokek Psoriasis Treatment Centre, The Galei Zohar Clinic and the International Psoriasis Treatment Centre (IPTC). All of them offer effective dermatological treatment for the skin.

## Climatological therapy

Only available at the Dead Sea, this successful treatment for psoriasis sufferers has become the most commonly recommended, natural, therapy by doctors, dermatologists and health care associations throughout the world. This treatment was pioneered, in the early fifties by the late

Professor Dostrowsky, and in recent years Israel has increasingly gained well-deserved recognition as a country where visitors can attend to their health, comfortably, enjoyably and under the finest medical supervision.

My personal experience of climatotherapy at the Dead Sea – 400 metres below sea level and the lowest place on earth – has shown that this unique, alternative way to restore your health, based on the climatic factors of the area, has been responsible, over the past twenty years for changing the lives of those who suffer and without doubt has proved to be a life saver to many.

The conducive climate of the Dead Sea region, one of the driest in the world, with high air temperatures and 330 sunny days a year are just a part of the natural curative factors that attract more and more psoriasis sufferers to Israel each year. Even in the middle of winter, days are warm and nights are pleasantly cool. Humidity is low (34-50%), atmospheric pressure high and rainfall sparse – rarely more than 50mm (2in) a year.

A unique haze hangs over the entire area, created by a high rate of evaporation. This is caused by the climatic factors of the Dead Sea. This haze contains large quantities of bromine, due to the high concentration of bromide in the waters of the sea, known to have a remarkable healing effect on the nervous system.

The additional layer of the earth's atmosphere at the Dead Sea and the haze that filters out the shorter ultraviolet UVB rays, while allowing the longer UVA rays to penetrate, means that very few cases of sunburn have been reported by the many thousands of visitors.

Scientists at Ben Gurion University of the Negev in Beersheba and the Weizman Institute of Science in Rehovat conducted comparative studies of UV spectral measurements of direct and scattered sunlight reaching Ein Bokek at the Dead Sea and Beersheba 280 metres above sea level. The two scientists obtained their results by using a UV meter and four filters which cut off light below 328, 357, 373 and 400 nanometres respectively. A comparison between the readings at the same time of day showed that the sunlight reaching Beersheba was at least twice as high in UV content as that reaching the Dead Sea. It also showed that the UV content of sunlight reaching the Dead Sea, in the erythema band (290-330 nanometres) was particularly low. It is not surprising that sunburn is extremely rare at the Dead Sea as erythema (reddening of the skin) is only produced by rays of wavelengths below 330 nanometres.

The waters of the Dead Sea are known for being one of the world's greatest concentration of minerals, providing raw materials for medicines, cosmetics, agriculture and industry. Virtually no multicellular organism or plants develop in the Dead Sea (in fact, a large lake) so called because of the extraordinary high salt and mineral content. The water is a concentrated solution of chlorides of calcium, potassium, sodium and magnesium and a high percentage of dissolved bromides. The salinity of the Dead Sea is 10 times greater than that of the Mediterranean Sea. The concentration of magnesium is known for its anti-allergic influences on the skin, is 15 times higher than in the oceans and the bromine is 50 times more concentrated in the Dead Sea than any other ocean in the world.

Bathing in the sea is very beneficial to sufferers of psoriasis and psoriatic arthritis, especially in severe cases where movement is limited, as the enormous concentration of minerals gives the water a high specific weight, which counteracts the weight of the body and allows you to float without any effort. This also is an ideal medium for therapeutic exercises.

Scientific investigation of the climatological treatment of psoriasis has taken place over many years, and the results have been that large groups of sufferers, regularly visit the Dead Sea, from the Netherlands, France, Switzerland, Italy, Austria, West Germany, the United Kingdom, Scandinavia, South Africa and America. Such has been the success of the treatment that government health authorities in Denmark, Germany and Austria pay all or part of the patient's expenses in those countries.

Private health insurance companies in Europe and now in the USA allow claims for climatological therapy. Sadly this is not the case yet in the UK.

An abstract from a research study by Dr David Abels and Dr Jonathan Kattan-Byron, both specialists in the field of psoriasis and climatological treatment, from the Division of Dermatology, Soroka University Hospital and Faculty of Health at Ben Gurion University of the Negev in Beersheba, serves to show you how the Dead Sea therapy may prove to be the right treatment for you too.

A naturally filtered ultraviolet spectrum of sunlight, along with other natural factors, is utilised in the management of psoriasis at the Dead Sea area in Israel. In 110 patients with psoriasis, 85.5% achieved complete clearance or excellent improvement. These results compare favourably with other therapeutic regimes used today in the treatment of psoriasis. Since systemic medications are avoided, the modality may be considered in the management spectrum of psoriasis.

Climatotherapy, defined as a treatment combining the natural elements of a specific geographical location, has been used at the Dead Sea for over 20 years. This study, one of many available, confirms the value of this treatment as a pleasant, natural way to relieve psoriasis, without the risk of unpleasant side-effects.

I have visited the Dead Sea many times, gaining my own personal experience of this remarkable therapy and I am convinced that the reason it is so successful is not just the climatic factors and expertise of the medical professionals, but at least half of the success can be attributed to the psychological benefits experienced by the sufferers.

These benefits are: feeling free to sunbathe without shame as the appearance of your skin at the Dead Sea is not a problem; watching your skin clear each day as you develop a wonderful tan and sharing your experience with others; making new friends and enjoying group therapy with sufferers from all nationalities and walks of life. Coupled with the opportunities of visiting tourist attractions, dancing, attending fashion shows, swimming, playing tennis, and pampering yourself by indulging in some of the latest beauty treatments. All those wonderful leisure and social activities are there to be shared with others who are convinced that clearing psoriasis at the Dead Sea is the right treatment.

If you are wondering, how long will you stay clear, after your return home, then the answer is that it depends on your general health and individual lifestyle. The average length of remission is between three and six months, but many cases have stayed clear for up to one year, and some for up to three years.

One young man from South Africa, on his fourth visit to the

Dead Sea, told me that his skin stayed clear from May until October after each visit, and his psoriasis returned less severely with less lesions each time. We discussed his everyday activities in his home environment and came to the conclusion that by re-adjusting his eating habits he could prolong his remission.

A patient from Europe reported that she had suffered from severe psoriasis since the age of 21 and was at least 80% covered with lesions when we met. For many years she had visited the Dead Sea for six weeks each year and successfully cleared her psoriasis each time. This allowed her to live a more comfortable life for a few months each year. She said: 'The Dead Sea has proved to be a life saver for me.'

A New York lawyer, who had visited the Dead Sea many times, decided to leave America and live in Israel in order to continue his life as a psoriasis sufferer near the Dead Sea, enabling him to relieve his condition at any time he chose. His psoriatic arthritis also cleared as soon as he had embarked on his new way of life.

A real estate agent from America, told me her story of how the Dead Sea had saved her life. Her condition was extremely severe as a result of many years of using drug-related creams and PUVA which had taken a physical, emotional and financial toll. After a few visits to the Dead Sea she decided that she would have to move to Israel in order to gain the quality of life she deserved.

Both these young Americans now spend their time helping others by introducing them to fellow sufferers and advising them how to enjoy their health treatment vacation.

I was asked to give group counselling to 20 South African psoriasis and arthritis sufferers who were visiting Israel for the first time. Naturally, their main concern, after clearing their condition during their one month stay, was how to stay clear for as long as possible when they returned home. They were given advice on self-care programmes, including diet and relaxation, which would help to prolong their remission times for several years.

Most of us cannot take a month's vacation – the normal time it takes to clear your skin at the Dead Sea – but I have experienced many cases who have cleared in two to three weeks. This is achieved by beginning your holistic education programme a few months before your health holiday.

A young man from India, had been a regular patient of the International Psoriasis Solarium for six years, staying for six weeks each time, as his psoriasis was very severe. His condition meant he was unable to gain employment so had to rely on friends and family to pay for his trips. This only served to create an added stress factor. The psychotherapist he had consulted for help, designed a programme of stress therapy techniques, and he began changing his eating habits five months before his departure. He was using the natural Pharbifarm range to alleviate his dryness and flaking. The result was that he cleared his condition in just two weeks.

Many sufferers ask why the health service in the UK does not contribute towards psoriasis treatment at the Dead Sea as some European administrations do. It costs the UK National Health Service £500 million each year to treat skin conditions by other orthodox methods.

## Mud therapy

As I mentioned before, psoriatic arthritis – that affects at least 5% of psoriasis sufferers, including myself – is also very successfully treated at the Dead Sea. Just one treatment at the Ein Bokek Clinic, famous for treating many rheumatic and arthritis patients for many years, cleared my arthritis. This is given under the expert care of exceptionally well-trained staff, and uses therapeutic mud from the shore of the Dead Sea, just north of Sedom. It is rich in salts and minerals from the lake, and also contains sulphides and bituminous products. The mud is capable of absorbing large amounts of water and is used in baths, wraps and spreads.

The thermo-mineral springs are also used in the therapy. This is known as balneological treatment, and the dissolved salts differ from those in the Dead Sea.

After being completely covered with the hot therapeutic mud and wrapped in a plastic sheet and towels for 30 minutes the mud is showered off, leaving the skin feeling smooth and comfortable. This is followed by immersion into the thermo-mineral bath. Unlike a normal bath, you float on the surface due to the high natural mineral content.

The heat of the water dilates the blood vessels and, as a result, circulation quickens and blood pressure decreases. According to research carried out by Dr D. Drugan, the human body is influenced by the dissolving mineral components in the waters in two ways (a) as a result of the influx and outflow of ions the equilibrium of the skin is charged, and (b) by the penetration into the body of certain mineral components.

# Chapter 3

# Alternative therapies that help

A few years ago, I was asked to present a paper, on Living with Psoriasis, at an international seminar in Spain attended by over 600 medical specialists from all over the world, including Russia, China, and Australia. Many of these people were also trained specialists in the field of alternative and natural medicine which they incorporated into the daily medical care of their patients.

One of the most remarkable people there was a lady from China, aged 93, who was a medical doctor and acupuncturist. She was presented with a golden key to a city in China for her contribution towards the health of her nation. Alas such accolades do not take place in the Western world so frequently. So what do we do in the meantime? We learn to take care of ourselves in the most effective, economical way possible.

Where do we start? My advice is to learn about the most effective natural therapies that will help your condition, with the emphasis very much placed on the word 'natural'. I have experienced many forms of alternative therapy and am convinced the key word in healing is 'self help'. Simple self-healing techniques, that are easy to learn, can be practised in your own home and become a way of life. Some of these techniques can be learnt from reading, but consultations with reliable alternative practitioners are recommended for more in-depth treatment.

I am not in favour with any treatment for psoriasis that depends on continued support from practitioners or medical professionals as I have seen many cases of despair when the condition returns or worsens after the sufferer has discontinued the prescribed treatment. Self-management, self-care, self-healing, self-help – they are the words associated with long-term health. I cannot emphasise enough the importance of the holistic approach to healing, taking care of 'all' your needs, and I hope that the following information, based on years of research for psoriasis sufferers in the field of alternative therapies will help you choose your own alternative way to suit your needs and lifestyle.

## Holistic medicine

This is a philosophy followed by the Hindus and Greeks thousands of years ago. The word 'holistic' means an approach to healing, not a medical practice, involving the treatment of the patient's individual physical, mental, spiritual and emotional needs. It uses the healing powers of nature and the self-healing powers of the patient. The patient and therapist share the responsibility of the illness.

The holistic approach to healing is a concept of natural therapy, known for helping to restore balance and harmony by healing the mind and body. This enables the body to release its own self-healing energy allowing the recovery of its own natural ability. A vital contribution towards the recovery of our health.

The South African philosopher Jan Christian Smuts introduced the word 'holistic' in 1926. In recent years it has allowed behavioural, humanistic and psychosomatic medicine to be combined, therefore helping to eliminate the more conventional practice of just regarding patients in terms of disease, the most common criticism of the medical profession. By spending more time helping the patient to deal with social, and personal problems – one of the reasons alternative practitioners are so popular – the patient is more able to make the necessary changes that will contribute towards a speedy recovery.

Dr Joseph E. Pizzorno Jnr, N.D., President of the Bastyr College of Natural Health Sciences in Seattle, Washington, USA, has been carrying out research studies using the holistic approach to stimulating the immune system in people with HIV, including lifestyle counselling, dietary advice, stress education using psychotherapy, and botanical medicine, and the results of his research were presented in the House of Commons, London, in June 1991.

## Homoeopathy

The practice of modern homoeopathy was established by Samuel Hahnemann early in the nineteenth century, whilst the principles originated from early medicine. Basically they are based on the premise of like curing like, with the homoeopathic remedy being matched to the substance that, if given in concentration to a healthy person, would produce the same symptoms as shown by the patient.

The intention is to trigger the body's defensive reaction therefore activating our natural resistance to disease. This is achieved by using minute homoeopathic doses of substances like sulphur, cadmium, gold, copper and a myriad other medicines, which go to make up the 3,000 available to the homoeopathic profession.

Homoeopathic therapy is designed to treat the patient, not just the disease. The mental, physical and emotional condition of the patient is taken into consideration during the first consultation. The patient's psychological pattern is also assessed to make sure they will suit the medicine recommended. Questions will be asked about, feelings, reactions, responses, needs and lifestyle, before the correct treatment is chosen. Reactions and symptoms that occur during the course of treatment should be reported to the homoeopathic doctor during the first few days and weeks of treatment. Choosing the correct remedy for the particular patient is a crucial part of the treatment.

A few years ago I developed a rash on my legs. It was not psoriasis. I was fortunate to be referred to an excellent young homoeopathic doctor from Greece, Dr A. Andrews, who prescribed the correct remedy after a lengthy discussion involving my personal responses and needs. The result was that my skin condition totally cleared within 24 hours and has never returned. This was my first experience of homoeopathic medicine but certainly not my last.

It is very difficult to understand why homoeopathy is successful with so many illnesses with the exceedingly small doses of medicine administered. There has been a great deal of discussion about the 'placebo' effect, but to disprove this homoeopathic therapy is also successful with animals. Just recently there was a documentary on UK television showing such a case. A homoeopathic vet demonstrated that a few drops of medicine added to the drinking water of cows had prevented the disease of mastitis developing, eliminating the need to inject the animals daily with drugs.

There does not seem to be any answer on exactly why homoeopathy works, despite a great deal of medical research being carried out. Many confirm that it works, but cannot explain why. Popular opinion is that it helps to stimulate our own self-healing process enabling us to eliminate disease.

Side-effects are almost unknown. A reaction is more common, particularly with skin disorders, as this form of treatment is known to bring the symptom outwards resulting in the condition appearing to worsen before improvement takes place. This shows the medicine is working, but it can be distressing to psoriasis sufferers. Hence the reason why we recommend that homoeopathy be used as a complementary treatment combined with the holistic education programme to gain maximum long-lasting results.

When consulting a homoeopath, first find out whether they are a medically trained practitioner or a qualified practitioner, and think twice about those who have just taken a brief correspondence course. A good homoeopath can contribute a great deal towards your health.

## *Naturopathy*

This therapy was founded by Hippocrates around 400BC. The principle of naturopathy is that all forms of disease are caused by excess toxins in the body, creating lack of oxygen, sluggishness and blocking our energy levels, therefore decreasing our self-healing process, affecting our body's ability to heal itself.

Many of these factors have been the case with patients at The Alternative Centre who, by changing their eating habits (the first advice a naturopath will give) have shown a considerable improvement in their energy levels and the condition of their skin.

Most naturopaths will recommend the elimination of foods that contain stimulants, like coffee, chocolate and alcohol, and some advocate the Hay System, that is, of not combining starch and protein together in the same meal. This dietary 'law' has proved for many to be one of the most effective ways to maintain good health.

The importance of a healthy way of living, with moderation in all things is the basic principle of naturopathy, and it can benefit us all.

## Osteopathy

Modern osteopathy was founded in 1874 by Andrew Taylor Still, and it is one of the forms of alternative treatment most readily accepted by the medical professional.

Known to be effective in the relief of backache, one of the most widespread complaints, this form of therapy can also deal with a wide range of problems, such as migraine, headaches, muscle tension, sports injuries and even stress conditions.

Cranial osteopaths are particularly good for releasing tightness of the head and shoulders caused by muscle tension and stress factors. This specialised form of treatment, pioneered by William Sutherland in the nineteenth century, has proved particularly helpful for psoriasis sufferers who are unable to consult an osteopath due to the lesions on their bodies.

## Acupuncture

Believed to have been practised in the Bronze Age about 3,000 years BC, acupuncture first became widely used in China. It is based on the principle that we are activated by an internal energy field, known as 'Chi', and as long as our energy flows freely disease cannot occur. The theory is that the body contains 12 main meridians along which our energy flows.

When any of the meridians become blocked, our energy decreases and we become ill. These are unblocked by placing needles, usually made from steel, into the identified acupuncture point on the body. There are over 1,000 points used in acupuncture treatment.

Once the needles have been inserted they are then delicately twisted, or pulled, to achieve the desired response, and left in place for a period of time. Sometimes very light electrical impulses are used. Patients should not feel any pain, but if pain is felt, as has been my experience, it is not unbearable.

In 1979 the World Health Organisation acknowledged that acupuncture could help a number of diseases. It has certainly helped patients with psoriatic arthritis by controlling pain and can improve lesions on the skin.

## Herbalism

This is one of the oldest of all the medicines and it also dates back to China some 3,000 years ago. Herbs have been used for centuries by man and animal, and many traditional cultures around the world practise herbal medicine that has been passed down through generations, and is part of their everyday life.

In China, professors of dermatology are trained in herbal medicine. This training takes many years as there are over 350,000 species of plants known to the herbal practitioners. These are prescribed after an initial consultation where the personality type of the patient is taken into consideration as well as the disease. The Chinese believe there are 12 pulses in the body, so rarely does a traditional consultation take place without the pulses being taken.

Individual herbs may be recommended or, more commonly, particularly with skin conditions (especially eczema), a combination of herbs are prescribed that may be taken as a tea, cream, poultice, used in the bath or made into a juice. Diluted, this treatment can be used for children and babies, under supervision. Many skin conditions have responded extremely well to this form of treatment, where other natural treatments have failed.

Herbs are a very powerful medicine and in some cases can be as toxic as drugs, often producing symptoms like nausea, indigestion, nervousness, headaches and giddiness. Anyone taking herbal medicine should not combine it with prescribed drugs and it is recommended that alcohol should be avoided as some treatments can cause a reaction. Above all, be sure you consult a well-qualified, medical herbalist before beginning any form of herbal treatment, as the correct prescription can help many of us.

## Massage

Massage has been practised for many thousands of years under many guises, some of which have been responsible for giving this valuable therapy a bad name. Massage, nevertheless, is without question one of the most therapeutic healing techniques today and can be enjoyed by many skin sufferers as they begin to heal. This therapy, with its physical contact, has a remarkable healing effect on those previously deprived of normal physical contact because of the condition of their skin.

As well as relaxing the muscles, therapeutic massage stimulates the blood flow, relieves pain, eases tension and increases the oxygen in the body. The neck, shoulders and back, where tension accumulates leaving us stiff and uncomfortable, respond to most types of massage therapy.

Massage combined with the use of essential, aromatic oils – a traditional form of healing developed in Europe after the Second World War by Marguerite Maury and her husband – also has a relaxing effect on the mind.

Kate Alden-Smith, specialist in therapeutic massage and aromatherapy, combines Western massage with Eastern pressure point techniques, and her treatment consists of massaging various essential oils, (carefully selected specifically for the patient) into the back, neck and down the spine, and the treatment is normally finished with a foot massage.

Two areas in which Kate's expertise has helped our sufferers at the Centre are with head and neck massage which aids the relief of tension and increases the oxygen supply to the brain and lymph drainage system, which in turn has an excellent healing effect on the autonomic nervous system. This is achieved by using a gentle rhythm technique that accelerates the lymph flow. At the same time a soothing effect on the sensitive nerve endings of the skin is achieved, with an accompanying reduction of sensitivity to pressure which can lessen pain for psoriasis sufferers.

Another area of Kate's work has been using massage in hospitals. This idea was pioneered by Clare Maxwell-Hudson, with whom Kate trained, and at Charing Cross Hospital. Working in close consultation with patients, massage proved a very effective treatment for patients with problems arising from stress and fatigue, reducing blood pressure and promoting a sense of well-being.

Kate says: 'During my work with heart patients at Charing Cross Hospital in London, the introduction of massage, as part of a scheme to reduce stress and improve the health of those with various heart conditions was responsible for the rehabilitation programme of patients who were suffering from a severe deterioration of health.

'The effect on the physical appearance of a patient who has regular massage is very noticeable. The skin tone and colour improves, especially noticeable in the facial area, leaving the patient looking younger and more healthy.

'My more recent work with skin sufferers has lead me to discover that the pure physical contact involved in massage and aromatherapy, and the feeling of relaxation that occurs after the treatment is complete, is without doubt a necessary part of the holistic healing programme for skin sufferers. By feeling good they begin to look good and this is where healing begins, in the mind.'

## Healing

The origins of healing go back far beyond Christianity. In ancient Egypt, the sick would lay at the feet of the healers – the priest and priestesses who practised natural medicine in those days.

There are very many healers in the world. Some practise absent healing, either individually or in groups, transmitting collective thought and energy to those in need. Others practise hands-on healing, coming into physical contact with the parts of the body that are affected by illness. The heat of the energy force, is quite often felt by the patient, although some have reported feeling cold during a session. Many healers just place their hands over the patient.

There are two types of healing. The first is spiritual healing where the healer transmits healing energy from himself to the patient, often without the patient's knowledge. The second is faith healing involving the patient and healer's energy and power being combined in such a way that the patient trusts the healer to make the best use of his or her body's self-healing energy.

Toni Simmons, spiritual healer, says it is possible that healing stimulates the self-healing hormones. It is particularly helpful when the patient does not have enough energy to use his own self-healing powers – a very common problem with psoriasis sufferers and others with chronic illness. Healing is a beneficial complementary therapy that can be used alongside medical and alternative treatment. It is one of the rare therapies recognised by our national health service allowing it to be used in hospitals. My personal opinion is that if you feel it will help you cope with psoriasis, don't discount it until you have tried it, as it certainly can help. Recent scientific studies by a medical team at Stanford University, USA, showed a measurable difference in the blood chemistry of patients who had received healing.

## Iridology

This is a diagnostic skill, founded by a Hungarian, Ignatz Von Peczley, in the nineteenth century. He designed the first iris chart used for diagnosis. The theory behind the science is that the iris of each eye is divided into 12 sections, each being related to five to ten parts of the body. Your health problem is transmitted and imprinted onto the iris. It is particularly useful in that this therapy can spot pre-determined health problems before they occur, allowing the patient to take preventative therapy.

I consulted London iridologist, Adam Jackson, not mentioning that I had very recently had a complete health check-up. By using a special microscope and sophisticated camera equipment, with no previous discussion on what my health problem could be, my diagnosis proceeded. The analysis showed, after reviewing the complex markings on the computer screen, almost the same conclusion as my previous check-up.

Iridology is a very similar diagnostic technique to Mora-Therapy, more widely used by doctors and hospitals in Europe, and to my mind is particularly helpful in terms of preventive medicine. Psoriasis sufferers are able to gain an in-depth knowledge of their general health problems that could be affecting their skin.

## Hypnotherapy

In practice this therapy began in Vienna in 1766 with an Austrian called Franz Anton Mesmer, although interest in hypnosis goes back centuries to early Egypt.

Such was Mesmer's success that he was banished from Austria by the medical professionals. He then moved to

France, but was again eventually asked to leave, despite the French King Louis XVI being an avid supporter.

For many years hypnotism has been associated with stage acts and evil practices, this having a damaging effect on its reputation as an effective therapy. Fortunately, over the past few years its benefits have become more widely accepted. It is now practised most commonly by psychotherapists, psychologists and psychiatrists, as well as doctors and alternative medical practitioners.

It can be very helpful for those suffering with addictions, phobias, eating disorders, stress related conditions, anxiety, and personal problems such as lack of confidence, fears, and pain control. It can also be used to delve into the unconscious mind to release past memories giving the therapist a lead in finding the cause of a patient's condition.

Hypnotherapy is often used with psychotherapy by Kenneth Wingrove-Gibbons, a specialist in skin conditions and renowned for his success in treating patients suffering from psoriasis. He says: 'Hypnotherapy is one of the most effective therapies for teaching the patient to relax and control their stress, and can very easily be taught as a valuable self-help therapy.'

Unfortunately, it is very difficult to assess who is a good therapist, since as it has become so popular it has also become very easy to become 'qualified' by taking correspondence courses with little practical experience. A referral by someone qualified in the field of psychology or your general practitioner can usually be relied on.

I have seen personally the way hypnosis has helped many psoriasis and psoriatic arthritis sufferers by enabling them to relieve pain, control itching and irritation, deal with the stress factors involved with these conditions, deal with insomnia and uncover the cause of the onset of their condition. But, probably most important of all, it has helped them, with the power of suggestion, to become more confident, a vital ingredient in the healing process.

## Autogenic training

A discovery in the nineteenth century of a self-hypnosis technique for stress control by two scientists named Brodmann and Vogt from Berlin.

The theory is that it is the patient's own healing ability, enhanced by calming and relaxing routines whilst in a semi-hypnotic state, that is responsible for the success of this treatment. The technique is to repeat positive affirmations related to your body, until the effect is felt, then the next affirmation or message is repeated and so on.

An example for psoriasis sufferers would be:

> My skin is comfortable
> My blood is cool
> My heart is warm
> My body is beautiful

As a staunch advocator of self-help therapies, which can be used without the support of a practitioner, I consider the positive effects of autogenic training – encouraging relaxation and promoting self-healing – to be invaluable.

## Auto-suggestion

The key to self-help and self-healing, pioneered by Emile Coué (1857–1926), a French chemist who is remembered for the phrase 'Every day, in every way, I am getting better and better.' Auto-suggestion can help patients overcome all physical and mental disorders as a result of stimulating their imagination, a concept along the lines of the power of positive thinking.

It is an excellent way of overcoming negative attitudes and despair, as it helps to re-programme the mind towards a more positive self-help approach to healing. The power of suggestion is not a new concept in healing and has been practised by many people, with excellent results, who want to achieve a more rewarding life. It is another simple, effective technique for you to practise, that will bring you another step closer to restoring your health.

## Meditation

Meditation, an ancient therapy, was first investigated and researched in the early 1970s by scientists worldwide. It has been established that you can become relaxed, rested and relieve stress-induced disorders by using this form of therapy. Research has also shown that blood pressure falls, the heart rate can slow down and anxiety and depression can lift.

Eastern mystics have been known to temporarily stop their hearts through deep meditation.

The world of meditation and its concepts are derived from centuries old practices of the East, linked with mystics and religion. It is an alternative way to deal with stress by triggering the body's own natural relaxation response. Meditation is a visual exploration – the attuning of the mental and physical body to its spiritual force. Meditation processes can change our own desires by taking us on an inner journey.

Thoughts stored in the unconscious mind can work against the desire of our conscious mind. For example, fear can be due to past memories. To rise above this we must re-programme our unconscious mind. Fear is responsible for mental disturbances – it is the root of all hang-ups which can result in physical illness. To release fear we must replace it with positive programming, trust, love, peace, positive concepts of self-image.

For most of us it is difficult to just relax. To allow ourselves to unwind can bring on feelings of guilt. To make time to soothe our minds is very important to maintaining our health. It is one of the self-help therapies I teach the patients who consult me, and I have seen some encouraging changes in both adults and children who practise this therapy for at least 30 minutes a day. Believe me, it works. I have used meditation as part of my healing process for many years.

## *Visualization*

Visualization techniques have been practised as a complementary therapy for many years, with some success with cancer patients. One of whom comes to mind is a young lady of 22 who was diagnosed as suffering from a growth in the stomach. Doctors in London announced that it was only possible for her to survive if they operated immediately, even then her chances were slim. Her parents decided to send her to a special centre in California where she was taught visualization therapy which she practised each day for a period of three months. On her return to London, she went for a medical check-up and was told there was no sign of cancer in her body and the growth had disappeared.

It is well known that our imagination can be constructive or destructive. Visualization therapy allows the mind to enhance the natural healing ability of the physical body. By changing the inner attitude of our mind we can alter the outer aspects of our lives, enabling us to control our destiny and safeguard our health. Our minds can make us ill; they can also make us well.

I first practised visualization for healing some twenty years ago, in an attempt to clear my psoriasis, and it worked. Each day I imagined that my skin was clear and that an invisible 'friend' was eating the red, flaking skin from the lesions on my neck. I consciously ignored the psoriasis patches when applying treatment. To my amazement, my patches cleared in six weeks. It may not work for everyone, but my results were successful.

Visualization therapy is very easy to learn and carry out on a daily basis. Don't discount it until you have tried it, as it can contribute towards clearing your skin.

## Colour therapy

Research at the University of California concluded that certain colours can help some patients. Experts like Theo Gimbel and Max Luscher are convinced that the power of colour has a great influence on our lives.

Some psychologists and medical professionals believe that personality can be assessed by our choice of colours. Hospitals have been experimenting on the use of colour for its healing effects on patients recovering from operations. The growing amount of evidence produced shows that we are all affected by colour. For years commercial industry has been selecting their colours for marketing strategy. Red is said to stimulate the appetite. Think of all the fast food chains. Green and yellow is associated with health.

What makes us choose the colours we wear? Observing the colours people wear can give us a clue to someone's state of physical and emotional health. Colour influences our lives and is more powerful than many of us realise. Some colours help in times of stress, others increase tension.

Yellow is important for the nervous system. For the skin it has powerful healing properties and it stimulates the mind's reasoning powers. Green is the colour of balance and harmony. Psychologically green brings a feeling of renewed freshness and brightness, like the colours of spring. Blue is light, cooling and relaxing and is associated with peace of mind. Violet has soothing and tranquillizing effects on frayed nerves, particularly with those who are nervous and highly strung.

There are many books on the subject for you to read, and for relaxation therapy associated with colour healing I recommend you buy a tape called *The Healing Rainbow* by Lilian Verner-Bonds, a well known specialist in this field.

My observation of psoriasis sufferers and the colours they choose has proved interesting. Many choose dark colours: browns, greys, and black. It appears that an attempt is being made not to draw attention to themselves. As their condition begins to improve they often introduce more colour into their make-up, hair and clothes, in the case of female patients. More often than not they are not aware of the psychological benefits of colour.

An experiment was carried out a few years ago by two specialists from America, with the blind. They were taken into a room painted red, wired to an electrical impulse machine to monitor the reaction of the body. Immediately, the volunteers showed agitation. They were then taken into a room painted blue, which showed a calming down effect on the body.

The influence of colour in our lives should not be overlooked as it does have an enormous psychological effect on our health.

## Art therapy

This has been practised for many centuries and has become accepted by doctors in hospitals for its valuable contribution to in-patients. An effective stress-release therapy, like so many creative activities, it allows the person to escape into a world of their own, express anger and frustration, and to restore energy. This form of self-expression therapy, as many psoriasis sufferers have confirmed, allows them to free emotions they are normally unable to express.

One artist, from Europe, told me that often she would paint all night long, explaining how the painting changed in terms of colour, depending on how she was feeling. She went on to add that it was the only time she felt totally free to express her emotions, and it made her feel very happy. The effect on her skin was noticeable and in her case art therapy has helped her cope with her psoriasis.

Creative energy, if not expressed, can affect your health. How many times have you wanted to attempt writing, poetry, drawing, painting or any other forms of creativity? According to my research the answer is, often. Do not wait for someone else to encourage you, and do not fear being judged, or make excuses that you do not have the time. Just do it. Believe me, it is a wonderful feeling of self-expression and stress-release.

## Bach flower therapy

Bach flower therapy is based on the philosophy that disease is a result of a conflict between the soul and the mind, and that it has to be treated spiritually and mentally to reach the primary cause. Treating the body alone just superficially repairs the damage, and cases of apparent recovery can be harmful since the root of the trouble is merely hidden. A good explanatory book on the therapy is *Heal Thyself* by Dr Edward Bach (C. W. Daniel).

## Music therapy

Music therapy was used for healing thousands of years ago by doctors in India during surgical operations. Now it is possible to take a degree in Music Therapy at the Catholic University in Washington. Thankfully it is becoming more recognised for its contribution in health care in Western society.

Music has been known to bring people out of a coma, when all else has failed. It can relieve pain and tension, restore energy, make you feel happy or sad, and for psoriasis sufferers it helps to alleviate stiffness of the body. It can also lift depression. Specialists in music as a therapy will confirm that the vibration of different musical instruments affect the body. The piano and strings combined appear to have the most relaxing effect. I recommend them for use with meditation.

It is easier to 'lose' yourself to the music of your choice by using a portable cassette recorder with ear phones, taking care not to play the music too loud, as this can affect your hearing. It can be used when travelling by plane, bus, train or when a passenger in a car. Be sure to always keep it nearby as it is an important means of self-healing and a wonderful way of controlling stress.

Many skin sufferers have confirmed that it helps them to cope with irritation. As a pain-control therapy it can work wonders, especially if combined with meditation. Music therapy must be classed as an essential part of our self-nourishment in our quest for good health.

## Voice production therapy

Voice production is another wonderfully effective therapy. Workshops are run by Chris James, one of the best teachers of this therapy in the world. Along with renowned musician Tim Wheater, Chris is performing in concerts in various countries to the benefit of many who find solace in his rhythms and sounds.

## Dance therapy

Also used for centuries, and in my opinion one of the best forms of physical exercise, especially for psoriasis sufferers, who tend to be too shy to go swimming or join a sports or health club.

All forms of dancing are beneficial, although one of the most enjoyable and effective I experienced, which involves the movement of every part of the body (and traditionally an artform that also exercises the mind) is Egyptian dancing. This rather sensual, colourful dance technique encourages the student to move gracefully and gently, improving posture and self-image.

Physical exercise is important to us all and something that is often last on our agenda. Most health clubs are expensive to join, so consider dance therapy as an alternative way of keeping fit.

## Psychotherapy

Psychotherapy treats the mind without drugs, and is a widely accepted complementary therapy that is endorsed by the medical and alternative field. Many doctors have trained in this therapy and it is widely used in the treatment of many ailments.

This form of psychological treatment and counselling helps in the treatment of shock, emotional stress, bereavement, divorce, anger, frustration, anxiety, addictions, phobias, eating disorders. It releases trauma and helps with the relaxation and stress release process so necessary for healing. It is a very important part of the holistic approach to illness, and has been used very successfully with many psoriasis sufferers.

The practitioner is able to offer a wide range of useful 'tools', in terms of auto-suggestion and expert counselling, which gives the patient the confidence to make the necessary changes in their lives that will improve their condition. They are able to reduce tension, give reassurance and encouragement, help the patient cope socially, lower emotional tension and deal with all the other emotional responses that affect the skin.

Some of the physical symptoms such as itching and flaking can be lessened by treatment with psychotherapy. It is a valuable aid to controlling stress. It offers the opportunity to learn a new more rational approach to dealing with the every day problems psoriasis presents. Most important of all, it teaches patients how to conserve their energy. Psoriasis sufferers carry with them a great deal of tension and this has to be released before progress in any form of healing can take place.

For keeping up to date with research and international news in the world of natural health care it is well worth reading the *Journal of Alternative and Complementary Medicine*, Mariner House, 53a High Street, Bagshot, Surrey, England GU19 5AH.

# Chapter 4

# Conventional medicine

If psoriasis is to be treated effectively, an understanding is necessary by the medical practitioner of the extent of the psychological stress associated with it, and careful consideration should be given to the highly toxic drugs that may have been prescribed.

In a recent report it was estimated that the average family doctor in the UK has 225 contacts with patients presenting skin complaints each year. That, of course, includes all skin complaints, just a percentage of whom are psoriasis sufferers. By far the majority of psoriasis patients in the UK are handled by their general practitioner, since there are only just over 200 dermatologists for a population of 58 million. By contrast Sweden has around 600 dermatologists for a population of 8 million.

These figures will help you understand why alternative medicine has become increasingly popular in many developed countries as an alternative way to treat psoriasis.

Before selecting the right treatment the correct diagnosis must be made and it is important that this should be made by your family doctor or a dermatologist as many alternative practitioners are not qualified in diagnosis, and wrong treatment can be recommended.

The second important factor is to fully understand the risk and benefit of any treatment prescribed, whether it is conventional or alternative medicine. These two factors, along with the following information on high-risk and risk-free treatments commonly recommended, will help you make the right choice.

The most widely used are coal tar, Dithranol and topical corticosteroids. In the UK these are standard treatments given by the general practitioner. Methotrexate, retinoids and PUVA, the more serious systemic drugs are left to hospitals and clinics.

## Tars

Coal tar is obtained as a by-product of the distillation of coal and is widely used for the treatment of psoriasis. Coal tar, in conjunction with ultra violet light, first used in 1925, is still the standard treatment used at the Mayo Clinic in America.

Wood tars, used in some preparations for the scalp, are said to have an antipsoriatic activity but are more irritating to the skin. This substance comes from trees with a high content of resin – principally pine and juniper. Hard wood tars come mainly from birch and beech.

The smell of the tars is very unpleasant, as many of you will know, particularly the treatment prescribed for the scalp which is also unacceptably messy to use. Many coal tar shampoos are recommended but, not surprisingly, have very little effect.

## Dithranol

Dithranol, or Cignolin, as it is known in Europe, and Anthralin in the USA is a synthetic derivative of a crude drug chrysarobin which occurs naturally in some plant extracts. It has been the mainstay of topical treatments for psoriasis for over 65 years, even though patients intensely dislike using it for the following reasons:

(a) It creates a brownish purple staining of the skin.
(b) Bandages are required, and clothes and bed clothes become ruined as the stains cannot be washed out.
(c) Bath staining, even bleach cannot remove.
(d) It causes irritation and burning-off of the top layer of skin if the strength is not carefully controlled, especially red haired or blonde people who easily burn in the sun, or those with pustular psoriasis. Irritation can also be caused to the eyes and mucous membranes.

A new Dithranol stick, as opposed to the more general use of pastes, pioneered in Finland, makes application easier and controls the mess to some extent. Short contact therapy is becoming more widely used and is said to lessen burning and irritation.

High strength Dithranol application is only used in hospitals. Pre-treatment with ultra violet light is said to help prevent after-effects.

# Corticosteroids

Corticosteroids are synthetic versions of steroid produced by our adrenal glands. Many sufferers are familiar with this treatment since it is easy and clean to use with no smell. Hydrocortisone is the milder of the group but has little effect on psoriasis. Dermovate, Betnovate, Synalar and New Budesonide are much stronger.

Topical steroids are easily absorbed into the bloodstream. Use should only be allowed for a short time but many patients obtain repeat prescriptions for years. With known side-effects and frequent non-effectiveness, warnings against use for psoriasis have been issued by clinical authorities. In my experience dermatologists prescribe this form of treatment less than doctors, although a study in Denmark indicated that in that country dermatologists used corticosteroids in 57% of cases.

The visible effects on the skin include thinning to the point of transparency, increased bruising, flushing, stretch marks, rashes and acne. It can also sometimes produce a fine downy hair growth on the skin. Oedema commonly occurs through the body's retention of excess sodium.

High-dose corticosteroids, used to suppress inflammation, interfere with the body's normal healing process and can lead to infection, and in extreme cases can cause skin ulcers. It is also known that there is a danger of getting high blood pressure and a type of diabetes. Prolonged use can lead to advanced osteoporosis because of stifled calcium absorption. Lowered potassium levels are known to leave muscles weak. They burn up Vitamin D and flush out zinc. They fool the body into producing less natural steroid, including one vital hormone, hydrocortisone, which we need to help us cope with stress. We know, without doubt, that stress control is an integral part of the healing process.

Because of the suppression of the body's ability to manufacture its own natural steroid, a long-term user of corticosteroids must be weaned off them gradually under the careful supervision of a well-trained health care professional. Most steroid creams are not recommended for use on the face, but are often prescribed for this.

Children especially should not use them as their skin is much thinner. If too much is absorbed, it is possible it will interfere with the growth of the child. Cases are often heard of children and babies being given these treatments.

## Methotrexate

Methotrexate has been used since 1955, and it has become a standard systemic drug to treat psoriasis. It is probably best known for its use in the treatment of various types of cancer, including leukaemia and Hodgkin's disease. It is also sometimes used to reduce the risk of kidney rejection after transplant. Because there is a recommended tolerable dose, which is normally over 3-5 years in order to avoid hepatic fibrosis or cirrhosis, it is, in theory, limited to older patients. Annual liver biopsies have to be undertaken and the complete avoidance of alcohol. It is said that most of the drug is excreted by the kidneys. However, it is recognised that 'some remains for weeks' particularly in the liver and kidneys. Not surprisingly, studies show a relationship between methotrexate and liver disease.

Not only liver and renal abnormalities are shown, but it is a folic acid antagonist and potent inhibitor of enzymes necessary for DNA synthesis. It is known to activate hepatitis and peptic ulcers, affect the blood cells of bone marrow, irritate the stomach and bowels and cause abnormalities.

It is now advised that appropriate steps should be taken to avoid conception during MTX treatment and for one year after its discontinuation. Other side-effects include nausea, indigestion, loss of appetite, abdominal pain, fatigue, dizziness, loss of concentration, mouth ulcers, skin ulcers, gastrointestinal ulcers, haemorrhaging, immune depression and hair loss.

Despite all this, however, a report from the Department of Dermatology, The Medical School, Chicago, Illinois, USA shows that MTX remains the best treatment for acute generalised pustular psoriasis resistant to topical therapy. PUVA is probably equally effective and safer, but less convenient and more expensive. They go on to say: 'No other established cytotoxic drug can challenge MTX and it retains a central role in the management of severe psoriasis.'

Sometimes, though fortunately rarely, Methotrexate is also prescribed for severe psoriatic conditions of the nails.

# Retinoids

Tigason, a brand name for Etretinate, a drug related to vitamin A, is most widely used. Roaccutane, the brand name for Isotretinoin, is also a vitamin A related drug.

Germany and Switzerland have been pioneering the clinical use of retinoids, but side-effects are holding back popular use. A statement issued by the Department of Dermatology, Free University of Berlin, Germany says: 'Compared with other methods of treating psoriasis, side-effects observed are numerous but mild, tolerable and reversible.' It goes on to list hair loss, severe gingivitis necessitating tooth extraction, an elevation of triglycerides and cholesterol, oedema, thirst, abdominal and musculoskeletal pain. In animal studies it shows an effect on cartilage tissue.

Patients can experience unpleasant dryness and irritation of eyelids and/or lips. Thinning of the skin develops, and there is increased fragility, itching, redness and peeling.

It is said that retinoids are not nearly as damaging to the liver as Methotrexate. Fetal malformation is the most serious side-effect. Since retinoids are stored deep in the tissues, they are detectable for many months after ceasing treatment. At this time Tigason can only be prescribed in a hospital or clinic since it is recognised that careful dosing and follow-up are needed.

One fact that is coming to light is that fat-rich food speeds the absorption rate of retinoids. I wonder whether dietary advice will be given, or taken into consideration.

# Razoxane

Used in Great Britain, this drug has now been withdrawn because of high risk of malignancy.

# Benoxaprofen

This has also been withdrawn from use due to severe side-effects, but the British medical authorities have approved a limited number of trials with psoriasis patients to continue.

# PUVA

Thousands of years ago the Egyptians treated psoriasis by eating an extract of weed which grows along the Nile and then exposed the afflicted area to the sun. It is also recorded as being used in India as early as 1500 BC for vitiligo.

PUVA is the modern version of this old technique and consists of the use of Psoralen, a photosensitizing drug, followed by UVA light treatment. PUVA use precipitates contact dermatitis, and in some cases it can become extremely severe. If the face is not covered during this treatment, facial eruption can occur within a few days of treatment. Patients often experience extreme nausea.

Pain and parathesia of the skin, in the form of a deep burning lasting from a few minutes to several hours, can either occur spontaneously following PUVA or can be provoked by scratching. In some cases this can be severe. There is a risk of cataracts of the eyes, and an eight-fold increase in the risk of cell carcinomas has been found in PUVA patients (Dept of Dermatology, Massachussetts General Hospital, Boston, USA).

During a visit by researchers from Stanford University USA to Peking Medical College, China, it was found that Psoralen has for several years been substituted with a Chinese herb *Angelica dahurica* which appears to have a Psoralen-like photosensitizing action. But, it is said, 'With minimum side-effects and greater safety.' I have not found anyone yet in the West willing to investigate these claims further.

## Peritoneal dialysis

Peritoneal dialysis has been used at the Warsaw School of Medicine, Poland, and in Germany on patients with extensive psoriasis. In trials about 30% of patients had a complete remission either during treatment or 2–3 weeks after its discontinuation. Regression of about 30% of lesions were observed in approximately 40% of patients. Despite only a slight improvement in the remaining patients (flattening of the plaque and/or 10-30% of the lesions) these patients were responsive to external treatment which was previously ineffective. This treatment is a standard method of removing waste from the blood of people with chronic kidney disease.

# Zinc

In a zinc tolerance test with zinc sulphate in psoriatic patients, from the Hadassah University Hospital, Ein Kerem, Jerusalem, Israel, zinc status was assessed in 12 patients with extensive psoriasis and compared to that of 11 healthy volunteers, using an oral zinc tolerance test. The 12 psoriatic patients were treated with zinc sulphate tablets 220ml×3 per day for three months and were followed up for an additional three months. A marked improvement was found in seven patients. All patients with psoriatic arthritis showed a good response to zinc.

**Note: We do not recommend you try this treatment without professional advice and supervision.**

## Sticking plaster

Even more intriguing is the use of sticking plaster. The following report appeared in *Options* magazine.

The Johns Hospkins University School in the USA discovered quite by chance that a plaster, or even ordinary sticky tape, placed over a patch of skin affected by psoriasis and left there for a week or so, improves the skin.

In the *New England Journal of Medicine*, a doctor describes how one of his patients with psoriasis, had a small piece of skin covered with plaster and it was not removed until three weeks later. Where the sticky plaster had been, the psoriasis had cleared. Surprised, the doctor applied sticky tape to other parts of the skin and the psoriasis disappeared from there too. More than a dozen patients were given the treatments with similar results.

The doctor speculated that the tape, keeping moisture and air out, stops skin cells multiplying too quickly. According to the doctor involved, Dr Shore, it worked better than steroid creams.

## Changing attitudes

A changing public attitude towards the medical professional and orthodox methods of treating disease has become evident in recent years as interest has grown in alternative, complementary and natural therapies.

Scientists and researchers throughout the world are very aware of the side-effects of some of the treatments they produce and are making an effort to curtail the manufacture of medicines that may harm patients, but it is important to understand that the drug-manufacturing industry is a very commercial and competitive business. Their sole function is to research, develop, test and market new treatments that will help to alleviate pain. The problem is that they tend only to treat the symptom not the cause, and many treatments cause toxicity during long-term use.

Note: There are many other conventional medical treatments available that are being used daily around the world, too numerous to mention in this book.

# Chapter 5

# About your skin

Our skin is one of the most extraordinary organs of the body, and it is a very efficient one. It protects us and constantly renews itself, and sheds dead cells. It eliminates waste, keeps our body temperature even, contains sensory organs which act as an early warning system, supports the growth of hair and nails, makes vitamin D from sunshine and provides a store of fat – all within a thickness of around five millimetres.

It is both waterproof and airtight, keeping harmful substances and moisture out of the body whilst controlling the loss of water and other substances from within. As well as depending for its health and well-being on the normal functioning of the body, it also has a very important relationship with the mind. Worry, grief, anxiety and emotional strain all take their toll.

The skin is made up of three layers, the top being called the epidermis, which in itself has four sub-layers. It consists of a horny covering of dead cells which constantly flake off. Underneath this covering, the living granular, prickle and basal cell layers are found.

The main function of the epidermis is to maintain and renew the protective horny layer. It takes about 28 days from the time a new cell is formed in the basal layer until it is shed from outside of the skin. The extreme toughness of this uppermost layer is due to the keratin, which also forms our hair and nails. It is kept supple by the secretion of various glands which have their openings in the epidermis. This helps protect the more sensitive lower layers against damage. The deeper layers are bathed in tissue fluid.

The basal layer consists of special cells which produce a brown pigment called melanin, which helps us tan in the sun. The dermis is completely different from the epidermis. It contains blood vessels, various tissue fibres, muscles, nerves, cellular elements and glands. It is the main part of the skin with the skin's blood supply running through the network of vessels ending in loops which return to the body's system of veins.

The sweat glands found in the dermis regulate heat by causing heat loss through evaporation of sweat on the skin's surface. Also in the dermis are the hair follicles – little pockets from which our hair appears. The nerve-endings of the skin are extensive and highly complicated. Nerve endings reach the dermis and are sensitive to heat, cold, itching and touch. It is in this role that our skin plays an important part in warning us of dangers; telling us what is hot, cold, wet, dry, smooth or rough.

Lymphatic vessels, which drain away protein substances, tissue fluids and the connective fibres, which bind the layers of skin together, are also contained in the dermis layer. There are, as well, elastic fibres (which give the skin its ability to stretch, as in pregnancy), and reticulan fibres, which ensure stability between the dermis and epidermis.

Finally, beneath the epidermis and dermis is the subcutaneous tissue which consists largely of fat. This acts as a protective cushion for the body, a heat insulator, and as a reservoir of fat for our body's various needs.

The physical reaction of our skin to what we are feeling psychologically is obvious. It turns pale when we are frightened; hot and red when we are angry or embarrassed. It secretes more sweat when we are anxious and it will tingle when we are excited. These reactions are normally involuntary and we have very little control over them.

When the various mechanisms go wrong, then our skin becomes the focal point of our attention and we don't take it for granted any more. There are many ways it can function improperly and cause one skin condition after the other such as in eczema, acne and dermatitis, to name but three. Psoriasis, of course, is one of the most commonly known, and is said to affect at least two per cent of the world population, but an eminent Professor of Dermatology from Stanford University in America suggests that three per cent could be more accurate: about 120 million people.

One investigation found the occurrence of psoriasis to be 2.85 per cent in 11,000 residents of the Faroe Islands. Another determined 1.4 per cent in over 39,000 people in five different regions of Sweden. Surveys have shown almost two million sufferers in the U.K., with new cases occurring daily. There are between four and six million in the United States, with 200,000 new cases each year. Australia has almost 500,000 cases, and New Zealand close to 100,000. Surveys in Japan and West Africa suggest it may be less common there, but it still affects a significant section of the population. A further 240 million may have inherited the tendency.

Despite these numbers and constant research being carried out around the world, less is known about the cause of psoriasis than any other skin complaint.

Psoriasis occurs in most races, but there are some exceptions. For example, in South America, research carried out on approximately 26,000 Indians, throughout 95 villages in Bolivia, Ecuador, Peru and Venezuela showed not a single case of psoriasis. Also, the true Aborigines of Australia had no record of psoriasis until they moved into Western society and integrated into city life. Popular belief is that whilst living in their original habitat they ate many natural plants, said to be high in vitamin C, as part of their daily life, and this may have been an important factor. Psoriasis is also rare in the Greenland Eskimo population, and it is thought to be based on their diet of cold-water fish known to be rich in EPA (eicosapentaenoic acid).

Sufferers from psoriasis have a hyperactive skin that appears red or dull pink and is covered in loose silvery scales that flake off constantly. This is due to the skin cells growing much faster than the cells of normal skin.

It can appear anywhere and everywhere on the body, including the scalp and nails, and there is often accompanying irritation. On the face it is uncommon and, fortunately, it is only in the more severe cases, many of whom I have seen at The Alternative Centre and at the Dead Sea, that the whole of the skin may be involved.

## Plaque psoriasis

This type of psoriasis affects by far the largest number – 95 per cent of sufferers. The basic symptoms are thin patches of red skin covered with dry, raised and crusted white scales. Lesions on both sides of the body often mirror each other. The epidermis, the outer layer of the skin, changes, causing increased water loss. As a consequence our skin loses much of its pliability due to the loss of body fluids which can escape three to ten times as fast as normal skin. Therefore, cracks can occur, particularly where the skin needs to be flexible on the palms of your hands and the soles of your feet. These same changes allow a higher percentage of penetration of substances coming into contact with the affected skin, which in many cases can worsen the condition.

There is an increase in the rate of the flow of blood which can result in reducing our body temperature, creating loss of energy, especially if many lesions are involved. This may explain why patches of psoriasis are red and bleed easily. The skin cells grow much more rapidly, every four days instead of the normal 28, seven times faster. The cells on the surface are still very new and more sticky.

## Other types

There are other types of psoriasis, such as guttate psoriasis from the Latin word *gutta* meaning drop. It looks like the skin has been sprayed with drops from a paint brush. Spots are quite small and there can be many of them. This form of psoriasis is more likely to occur following a sore throat or tonsillitis. It is rarely known to affect children.

Generalised psoriasis is red over the entire body but is less scaly than plaque psoriasis. In rare cases the water and heat loss can be severe.

There are two other conditions named as psoriasis that more recent research considers may not be psoriasis at all. First, pustular psoriasis, where pus spots occur more commonly on the palms of the hands and the soles of the feet. White spots develop which very quickly turn yellow, then brown and then disappear. Second, nappy or diaper psoriasis which, as the names implies, occurs especially in young babies.

Psoriasis of the nails more frequently affects sufferers from psoriatic arthritis. Five per cent of psoriasis patients have some form of arthritis, and five per cent of arthritis patients have some form of psoriasis. The joints are attacked at the ends of the fingers, and nail changes take place, believed to result from the same defects in the keratinization process as in the skin. The main changes in the nails are of three types. Pitting, separation of the nail plate and changes such as thickening and discolouration. Complete loss of nails can occur, but fortunately this is very rare and is usually only associated with very severe psoriasis.

Psoriasis can appear at any time during our life. Science suggests it is a genetically inherited weakness. In many cases members of a family have a history of psoriasis, arthritis, diabetes or gout, so a genetic link seems possible.

Whilst research has broadened our knowledge of the biochemical, pharmacological and genetic aspects of psoriasis, the exact cause remains elusive. There are many schools of thought on the subject. Some theories are that it could be caused by the herpes simplex virus related to chicken pox and shingles; too much cholesterol in the blood or liver; respiratory problems or faulty elimination causing toxicity in the system. Others include an imbalance of the central nervous system, an inefficient pancreas, or hormonal changes, a metabolic disorder, lack of a specific enzyme causing an inability to utilize fats, or perhaps an allergy to certain drugs, or food intolerances. So it goes on.

Research has shown that psoriasis can be triggered by varying factors. Some of these could be a respiratory infection, physical or chemical injury to the skin, or psychological stress such as exams, bereavement, divorce or perhaps a significant change in environment or lifestyle.

## Delayed onset

We know that psoriasis can take up to two years to show itself on the skin after an illness or trauma has passed. A TV Drama Producer experienced her first outbreak of psoriasis after a respiratory infection, at the age of 11. In another instance psoriasis first appeared when the young lady concerned discovered she was adopted. This occurred at the age of seven when she also had chicken pox.

Psoriasis began for one patient after being sexually molested at boarding school. A patient from Europe I interviewed during my research at the Dead Sea told me her condition first appeared after a miscarriage at the age of 21.

An eight-year-old boy became the only sufferer at school after his parents divorced. Another young girl of ten became a victim when her sister was born. The oldest case I have knowledge of was a lady whose husband had died causing her psoriasis to manifest itself at the age of 93.

These and many other cases confirm that the onset of psoriasis is caused by physical or emotional illness. All the influences of our life affect our skin. The food we eat, the liquids we drink, our choice of cosmetics, toiletries, washing powders, kitchen utensils, the air we breathe, water, sunlight, heat, cold and environmental and electro-pollution can all be a source of aggravation to our condition. Consider the side-effects of some of the drug-related treatments on the skin. The use of synthetic fibres and tight fitting clothing, known to increase irritation.

What about our levels of stress, tiredness, anger, frustration, sadness, negative thoughts? These influences, as with so many others can result in constant scratching causing damage to our skin. These factors do not cause psoriasis alone but our experience shows us that they can interfere with our ability to respond to treatment. Our skin is a reflection of what goes on in our mind and body and mirrors our own level of health.

The skin acts as a reflective surface for all our internal organs and shows us signs of degeneration taking place inside the body. Every disturbance is shown on the skin. It also signifies our psychological state, our sexuality, or receptiveness to touch and contact, it protects and separates us from contact and reacts when we are distressed.

Our skin reveals a great deal about what is going on in our mind. When it shows itself in the form of a rash, lesions or other visible symptoms we are actually letting go of something that needs to come out in terms of emotions. Psoriasis sufferers are victims of not letting anything in or out. The horny layer of skin becomes like a suit of armour, acting as a protection from anyone we perceive may hurt us. The bigger the fear which manifests first in our mind, the thicker the skin becomes, and the more sensitive we are the more we fear.

This protective coating does protect us, but it also prevents us from receiving and allowing in the most important thing of all, love and devotion from those around us. The one human emotion we all need the most is the one we try so hard to resist. By doing this we are depriving our soul from the joy of life. This is based largely on the fear of the unknown.

Once you begin to understand the 'healing power' of illness, and the analysis of symptoms and what causes us to become ill or suffer from a condition like psoriasis you are well on your way to restoring your health. This comes from honest self-assessment. The seeds for disease are sown in the mind, they then show themselves in the physical body alerting us that we have not recognised and dealt with the psychological and emotional factors affecting our lives. We are holding something in; normally the suppression of memories, thoughts, hurts, fears and a host of other psychological factors that cause us to react on a physical level. We have to experience the pain of letting go to be able to experience the pleasure. Fear of feeling, of intimacy, of being hurt, of being vulnerable; all these are symptoms of skin conditions. We suppress them in our mind and they have no choice but to burst out of our skin. When itching occurs with psoriasis, it is a symptom of something irritating you that is stimulating the thinking process. Something is bothering you, like an inner fire burning. Scratching is like digging into your skin, trying to eliminate something by uncovering it. Once you discover the cause you can dispel the symptoms.

Try looking into your unconscious mind, it can be very enlightening, see what it is that is creating this physical symptom of itching. What do you need to release – anger, sexuality, aggression, passion? What is getting under your skin? Somewhere you will find the solution. Understanding your mind and body and the influence each has on your health is the first step in your recovery programme.

# Chapter 6

# How to take care of yourself

Taking care of yourself is the most important aspect in a self-healing programme. You have to turn your attention onto yourself, something we are often unable to do. Mothers and wives who are psoriasis sufferers regularly say to me: 'But I cannot possibly find the time to relax and take care of *my* needs. I don't have time to have fun; I have to be with the children; they need me.' Time and again guilt prevents us from taking time away from others to take care of ourselves.

This is also a symptom of lack of self-love in that we do not feel we deserve to take time for ourselves for our own pleasure or well-being. We over-compensate in the care of others in order to gain love, to win the love we feel so sadly lacking from within. This comes from our own feeling of inadequacy at not feeling good enough. This is not just a symptom of having psoriasis, but goes much deeper than that. Some patients will not even consider making the slightest contribution towards themselves, which is a reason the normally prescribed drug-related creams are popular because some measure of relief can be gained without taking much time to take care of yourself.

These cases are very sad, and the sufferer continues to worsen their condition as the years progress. Men make the excuse that they are too busy and tired, which is of course one of the reasons we advocate food and therapies that promote energy.

The important factor to consider is that you are actually being more selfish by not making the time for yourself to restore your health. It is common sense that if you feel well, able to cope and your psoriasis is comfortable, in remission or under control, automatically the people around you will benefit. You owe it to yourself and others to make the time each day to follow all the recommended suggestions that will improve your health. One hour is about all you need; or even less once your skin begins to heal. It certainly saves you a lot of valuable time later.

## Taking care of your skin

Taking care of your skin is the first step, and easy-to-apply methods of doing this so that the minimal interruption takes place in your daily life have been practised by ourselves and many patients at the Clinic. Any substance that comes into contact with the lesions of your psoriasis can worsen your condition, so it is important to carefully check the ingredients and the effect they have on your skin, and to be aware of what you can do to prevent these uncomfortable reactions, which may be increased flaking, redness or itching and bleeding.

For example, washing powders are particularly abrasive if they contain enzymes and any biological substances and chemicals. This also applies to fabric conditioners which, to my mind, are totally unnecessary if you wash your clothes and household items in one of the excellent brands now available for sensitive skins.

I realised some while ago after accidentally adding a biological powder to the washing machine that fabric conditioners were only necessary to soften the clothes that had become stiff and impossible to wear or iron after being exposed to these abrasive detergents.

I know of a case of a young lady who had psoriasis on the face which appeared at irregular intervals, but was nevertheless embarrassing to her and seemed impossible, despite years of steroid creams, to remove permanently. After some detective work we revealed that she always took her weekly wash to the local launderette who, of course, used their own brand of washing powder guaranteed to make your washing very clean. After changing the powder to her own selected brand her condition cleared for the first time for nearly ten years. Abrasive washing powders will cause your skin to itch and flake more rapidly, so if you want to help your skin and protect those in your family we recommend two brands. One is Boots own-brand range of washing powders, liquid detergents and washing-up liquid and they have helped to bring relief to many sufferers.

I would like to add that one of the top executives at the Boots

Head Office approached us some years ago to ask how they could help in manufacturing a product suitable for all the skin sufferers who were besieging them (on our instructions). Thankfully they succeeded in producing a safe alternative to the more commonly advertised household names.

The other brand is called Ecover. They produce the same basic products as Boots but with the addition of a floor soap, hand cleaner and a cream cleaner for household all purpose use.

Frequently a patient will ask: 'Yes, but do they really get the clothes clean?' My answer is always: 'Of course, otherwise they would not be such a best-seller, and your skin is actually more important than the whiteness or the brightness of your clothes.'

Toiletries are another important consideration. Many claim to be for sensitive skins, detergent and additive free, but if you look closely you will see that deodorant contains aluminium. Not seriously to be considered as contributing towards our health, I hope. One brand we recommend which is normally available in the health stores is called Multiherb. If you need something stronger we advise you take Chlorella, a natural deodoriser in the form of a food supplement, as it contains a high amount of chlorophyll.

Toothpaste is another suspect product that can affect the body, so we recommend two brands containing no harmful additives, *Kingfisher* and *Sarakan*, both available at health stores.

The product names recommended above have been tested on many psoriasis sufferers using the Mora-Therapy technique and have shown time and time again to have no adverse side effects on a considerable number of patients. We test many products in this way, with patients recommended to bring their own favourite brands for testing, and we are constantly searching around the world for the best possible foods, products, treatments, supplements and books for our patients' health.

Soaps with perfume and colouring can cause irritation on the skin, and even the non-perfumed varieties, although good for sensitive skins, may not be suitable since psoriasis is not just sensitive skin. Soaps containing aloe vera extract, from a remarkable South American cactus plant known for its healing effects on burns and other skin conditions, are recommended, as is our own brand of *Pharbifarm* soap which was specifically developed for psoriasis sufferers.

Most shampoos contain detergent, which is why, I feel, so many of us suffer from dandruff. They are designed to take the grease out of your hair but they also succeed in taking it out of your scalp. Then we have to buy conditioners and anti-dandruff shampoos that can be very abrasive. However, psoriasis is not like dandruff, so don't expect these shampoos to clear your condition. I know they can prove helpful but they are abrasive, and as psoriasis sufferers lose their dead skin cells very much more often than normal these shampoos can actually aggravate your condition.

After many years of looking, the only shampoo we have discovered that does not harm your skin and worsen your scalp psoriasis is the *Pharbifarm* shampoo, available from The Alternative Centre, as are all the other *Pharbifarm* range of natural products, specifically developed in Sweden for psoriasis sufferers. It contains no colouring or detergent and is 100 per cent soluble.

The truth is that we have not had any psoriasis sufferers bring to our attention any other product that worked as well. It will not be able to clear your psoriasis without the No. 1 and No. 2 Formula, which has to be used every day for four weeks. Normally this length of time clears the condition, and thereafter, by continuing to use the gentle shampoo, you will help to keep it away. Many patients who have returned to their normal brand have reported that their condition returned very quickly.

For conditioners, natural henna wax has proved very effective and comfortable for the hair. For those of you who wish to tint or rinse your hair regularly (and personally I feel the result is worth a little suffering) just be sure to take your own shampoo and conditioner to the salon, as their commercial brands can be abrasive, although we are pleased to see that many more hairdressers are now using natural products for the hair. Don't be shy about explaining what is wrong with your scalp.

Keeping your hair shorter helps to eliminate the time spent with a hairdryer. Be sure not to hold it closer than twelve inches from your head and towel dry your hair before using the dryer. For those of you who want to perm your hair, the same applies as for colouring. Ask your hairdresser to recommend a gentle perm and try not to have one too frequently.

Brushing your hair before sleeping will help to eliminate irritation, and be sure to wear light colours so that the flaking does not show so readily. A bright coloured scarf helps as it can be shaken readily.

Cosmetics for the purpose of moisturising, make-up and cleansing should be carefully selected. Lanolin is one of the most common ingredients in these products and one which many people are allergic to. The most consistent one we have tested on patients is from the Marks and Spencer range 'Extracts of Nature'. Many of the Marks and Spencer products are excellent in the field of skin care and can be recommended.

For a moisturising lotion for the body, *Mill Creek*, an American brand available in health stores, has proved excellent. If your skin is not too sensitive you could add a little of your favourite perfume to your body, after applying the lotion. Alternatively dab perfume on your hair if your psoriasis will not allow it on your skin. For cosmetics for the face the *Clarins* range of products consistently tested well, although obviously quite expensive.

Shaving of hair, either for men or women, is best achieved with a wet shave and applying a non-allergenic moisturiser, or the *Pharbifarm* soap before shaving. In extreme cases of sensitivity, if the psoriasis lesions are on the shaving area, we recommend you apply a homoeopathic cream called *Traumeel* which is anti-inflammatory and available from The Alternative Centre.

If waxing is preferred for hair removal, it has been shown that cold wax treatment, now widely available in beauty salons and for home use, is preferable to hot wax treatment. A new sugaring technique used in Middle Eastern countries has proved exceptionally gentle on the skin.

For the bath or shower it is important to protect your psoriasis from the harsh elements of the water. This can be done by applying a moisturiser before you shower or bath, using a non detergent soap, and adding a bath product that will protect your skin, and not the more usual bubble baths that contains detergent. Some of the mineral salts baths are excellent, but be sure to shower immediately as they may cause your skin to itch.

We discovered that adding to the bath an essential oil, like lavender for relaxation, helps the skin. *Bodytreats* is a brand we recommend as they are excellent quality and value for money. They make a wide range of fragrances, all of which have different beneficial effects.

Another product to add to the bath that can help your skin is called *Mamina* from Mamina Springs in the Andes. This natural product, the colour of red clay (but it won't stain the bath), is a blend of soluble salts, containing magnesium, calcium, potassium, sodium, nitrogen, sulphur (used in homoeopathy for psoriasis sufferers) phosphorus, boron, zinc and many other trace elements. This combination of salts and trace elements helps to maintain the chemical balance of the body, which is vital for our health. This product has been used successfully in one of the leading hospitals in Chile for the treatment of various skin disorders, backache, general stress and rheumatic and arthritis conditions. It is almost like enjoying a spa treatment in your own home. It is available through The Alternative Centre by mail order for those of you who would like to try it.

The *Pharbifarm Bath Formula* has also proved successful over many years as a bath additive. It contains essential oils and extracts of plants that protect the skin from the water. Again, your favourite essential oil can be added to this formula.

Some patients have complained that the metal substances contained in jewellery can cause a reaction to their skin, especially if say a watch is worn near a lesion. There is a special clear substance that can be painted onto non-gold ear rings to help protect you from metal allergy – available from pharmacists. Leather straps for watches are more acceptable than gold or any other metal as the strap allows the skin to breathe. If your body is over-acidic because of your diet, you will experience a more intense allergic reaction on the skin. Good costume jewellery can be worn on clothes if you want to avoid jewellery coming into contact with your skin.

## Good grooming

Before we move on to the subject of clothes and fabrics may I stress the importance of paying attention to grooming. A great many psoriasis sufferers let themselves go, and this tends to make them look unattractive, and only serves to create the very thing they want to avoid; rejection. I know it is not easy to feel good when you wake each day with your skin problem, but making the effort to try to look good will really help you to want to get well.

Remember that you only see yourself for perhaps a few minutes each day in the mirror. It is others that have to look at you for the rest of the day, and we have a responsibility to look good for their sake as well as your own self-esteem. Not looking good, clean and fresh; not bothering to try to make ourselves acceptable and attractive leaves us feeling depressed, isolated, withdrawn and lacking confidence. Even just selecting some clothes in bright colours, a little lipstick and clean hair looks and makes you feel wonderful. It does not matter how hard we try, we cannot hide away just because we have psoriasis.

Don't be afraid to experiment, change your image, perhaps your hair colour or style, buy a wig, there are some marvellous ones around that look very natural. Choose clothes that are different from your normal style. All this is part of becoming the new you. It does not take a great deal of time and need not cost much money. You could even consider changing your name. You would be surprised how a new hair colour or style, some bright colourful clothes and perhaps a new name can help you to feel better about yourself.

## Clothes and fabrics

When selecting clothes be sure to choose those made from natural fibres, like cotton, silk and wool, as they allow your skin to breathe and will help to prevent irritation. This also applies to undergarments. Synthetic fibres cause your body to lose moisture which can increase flaking of the skin.

Bed linen should also be selected with this in mind – cotton sheets, pillow cases, natural fibre blankets – and be sure to avoid feather pillows and duvets. All these precautions will help you to achieve a good night's sleep, free from irritation. Taking an air bath before you go to bed with some gentle exercise, moving your arms and legs, allowing the air to circulate around your body, is another effective way to reduce irritation.

## Sleep

Sleep is a vital human need and every effort must be made to achieve a peaceful relaxing night's sleep. One third of our lives is normally spent asleep, and sleep deprivation is one of the greatest threats to our skin, and one of the commonest problems associated with psoriasis sufferers. Take a look at your skin when you next experience a peaceful night's sleep, you will see a difference, as it is during sleep that our skin cells regenerate, which is why psoriasis sufferers must make sure they sleep well.

A good night's sleep is associated with warmth and comfort. When we fall asleep we are surrendering ourselves. Those who suffer from insomnia are unable to surrender themselves; they lack trust and don't feel safe enough to let go. This could be because of fear or something irritating you, and in the case of psoriasis sufferers it is normally manifested in the skin. If you oversleep or have a problem waking, ask yourself what it is during the day that you want to avoid.

Sleep is nature's healer, as it gives the body and the mind time to relax and restore energy. This is why it is so important. Our body rests during sleep but often our mind is unable to. This is why sometimes we wake up feeling exhausted. There are a few simple aids to ensuring a good night's sleep.

Chamomile tea, or one of the herb teas especially for drinking at night time, are very relaxing and certainly help in promoting sleep. There are also some herbal sleeping pills available containing herbs that have a tranquillizing effect. These are not addictive, and are suitable for those of you who need something stronger.

Relaxing music or simple meditation to music works wonders if you just allow half an hour, in bed, to practise it. It is also very helpful if you wake up during the night because of irritation of the skin or worries. Just reach for your portable stereo with ear phones and your choice of meditation music, perhaps even one that has subliminal messages incorporated in the music, or alternatively the sound of the sea, and after 15-20 minutes you should be relaxed enough to resume sleeping. All this can be done without disturbing your partner.

This technique can help you if you wake up tired. Just allow 30 minutes before rising, set the alarm in case you fall asleep, and you will start the day refreshed.

The quality of sleep we get also depends a lot on our activities of the day. If you have accomplished something you feel is worthwhile and satisfying, this will leave you with a relaxed feeling. If you have left something undone or you are wrestling with a problem, you are more likely to be in a state of unrest, and this will inevitably lead to a restless night.

Eating late at night, an argument or something disturbing that you read or saw on the television, can stimulate your hormone production and keep you awake. This is a physical reaction of the body related to insomnia which as you can see has a chemical basis.

Noise, of course, is another source of disturbance to our sleep – perhaps a partner snoring, or traffic noise. If this is the case, try using ear plugs. Boots' ear muffs are a wonderful investment in a restful night.

Ideally we should wake each morning at a certain time without the aid of an alarm clock or early morning call. If we don't, then we are not getting enough sleep. Our sleep cycle should be controlled by our biological clock and not by artificial means.

Catnaps can be very valuable, and they are usually quite easy to achieve during the day. They have the effect of re-charging your energy by resting your mind and body. Just half an hour's relaxation with meditation is said to be the equivalent to eight hours sleep.

Too much sleep, though, can make you feel lethargic. So, what is the ideal amount we need? This varies, and I feel it must depend on the energy you need each day. In other words, it is the hours you are awake and what you have to achieve in those hours that determines how much sleep you need. Some of us need ten hours, others only five, but the average seems to be somewhere between seven and eight hours per night. I recommend that patients should aim for at least eight, as a great deal of energy can be used up with the stress factor of just being a sufferer. But remember, it is the quality not the quantity, and it does improve the condition of your skin.

It is interesting to know the process of sleep. First, we fall into the state between waking and sleep. Second, our brainwaves become longer and slower. Third, our brain waves slow down even more and our bodily functions are also affected at this stage. On the final stage we reach a state of unconsciousness. This gradual sleep inducement process takes about one hour.

Sleep helps to protect us from illness, as it helps improve our immune system. The most likely time to catch flu or a cold is when you are tired. If we don't get enough sleep our cells do not repair themselves fast enough.

One of the most important considerations for a good night's sleep must be your bed. Not only must it be comfortable, but it must be regularly aired to remove dust mites which can create allergy problems. Unpleasant as it sounds, they live on the dead scales of our skin and may be a reason why we itch during the night. Be sure to vacuum your bed mattress and air it regularly.

It takes patience and practice to be able to re-adjust your sleeping patterns, just the same as it does to re-adjust your eating habits, but it is worthwhile. There could be a reluctance to try if you feel it will affect your partner. Do not immediately impose your new regime on them if their body clock or needs are different from yours. You could try taking a nap or using meditation to regain your energy when you return home from a busy day. This will help you to increase your energy and lessen your need for more sleep.

It may in time be possible to encourage your partner to enjoy going to bed earlier. After all, earphones can be used for personalised music or be plugged into a television so you can enjoy separate activities. Be creative and try it.

I discovered some years ago the benefit of sleep to my psoriasis. After a particularly stressful phase in my life, which caused my condition to flare up, a doctor gave me an injection that put me to sleep for over 24 hours. I woke to find that my psoriasis had cleared from my skin.

## Hands and feet

Psoriasis sufferers with lesions on their hands and feet have a specific problem, and patients with psoriasis on their hands sometimes tell me of having been turned down for employment and of the reaction they have experienced when serving friends or family with food. Even receiving change while shopping can create an upsetting reaction. One young lady, employed as a secretary, told of her distress when her boss insisted on spraying disinfectant on the switchboard in the office after she had relieved the receptionist. His reason was that he was afraid the other staff would catch her complaint.

You must be sure to protect your hands from household products and other abrasive factors, just as you would the rest of your skin. This can be done by wearing gloves, whether you are gardening, doing home improvements or just household chores. It will protect your hands from chemicals, and also from the risk of cuts and abrasions. Put cotton gloves inside rubber gloves at all times otherwise you will create irritation. Prevent germs from building up inside the gloves by rinsing them thoroughly and letting them dry inside out. For the preparation and handling of foods, surgical gloves are excellent and available in most chemists.

The application of a moisturising lotion, the *Mill Creek* or *Pharbifarm No. 2* oil, before wearing gloves will ensure the minimum loss of moisture from your skin. Avoid water that is too hot, even with your gloves on. It is a sensible idea to carry the soap you are using with you so you avoid the risk of having to use soap unsuitable for your skin.

For social events invest in a nice pair of gloves, or for special occasions perhaps long evening gloves.

For your feet use comfortable leather footwear with leather soles and low heels. This will help your skin as the leather allows it to breathe. For sports or gardening a pair of cotton socks will help if you have to wear footwear from synthetic materials.

One patient reported a problem with her feet which seemed to worsen after time spent at a horse stables, and which had become so severe she was almost unable to walk to the clinic. We discovered that for as many as eight hours per day she was wearing rubber boots which were causing her feet to perspire, and the result of the continual loss of moisture was that her skin was flaking very rapidly causing her feet to become inflamed and very painful. It was recommended that either she purchased leather boots or cotton socks to solve the problem that was preventing her from carrying out her job.

Hand and foot psoriasis is most commonly associated with a problem in the kidney area, and is one of the most stubborn forms of psoriasis to deal with. It is also one of the most disabling and painful, but it can be treated with some success.

Sometimes the materials that your skin comes into contact with can cause the condition to become more severe. One patient was in contact every day with aluminium at the aircraft factory where he worked. Another was affected by the chemicals used in the ink for printing newspapers. Building workers who come into contact with cement are also vulnerable.

Psoriasis of the nails is often a symptom of a tendency to arthritis. This can be helped with a change of diet, but one of the most successful remedies we have found for this particular condition is oil of marigold, applied to the nail every day for about six months. Marigold flowers have become well known for their healing properties, and form the basis of creams, lotions and a number of skin care products available in health stores. They are also used in homoeopathic medicine.

Dr Mohammed Taufiq Kahn, a homoeopathic chiropodist who practises privately and at one of the London hospitals, was responsible for the research that revealed that marigold treatment is good for psoriasis of the nails. You have to be very patient as it can take at least six months to work, but as this condition is also cosmetically unattractive it is well worth persevering. It is available from The Alternative Centre.

Here are some further useful hints which are worth considering as this condition is not a pleasant or easy one to deal with.

Keep your nails short, but make sure you soak them in warm oil, like almond oil (available from chemists and health stores) or *Pharbifarm No. 2* oil, a few minutes before cutting; and use a good pair of nail clippers, not scissors.

On no account expose them to any abrasive chemical products, cleaning materials or water.

Drinking half an ounce of gelatine stirred into water each day, without fail, promotes the growth of new nails and improves the condition of the nail bed. (Kosher gelatine is available for those of you not wanting to take the normal product.)

## Smoking

I would like to draw your attention to the subject of smoking and its relationship with your skin and your health, but I am not going to go into the dangers of smoking in detail as I am sure most of you who do smoke are already aware of them. Many patients ask us if giving up smoking will help their psoriasis. It will not necessarily directly help your psoriasis, but it will contribute towards your health and the health of those around you.

What most of us are unaware of is that smoking not only

depletes valuable vitamins from our body but causes premature wrinkles on our faces especially around the mouth and on the forehead. For some of us the thought of prematurely ageing is more of a deterrent than the risk of a life-threatening disease.

Think about the damaging effects of smoking on your health, which I promise you will occur one day. As we are subject to so much harmful environmental pollution, most of which we are unable to avoid, the effects of tobacco smoking on your lungs are even more dangerous to your health than they may have been many years ago.

If you want to make a commitment to give up cigarettes there are ways to make it easier. One way is to convince yourself how ridiculous it is to put a roll of chopped leaves in your mouth and set light to them. Another is to put the money into a glass jar everytime you want to buy a packet of cigarettes. You can help yourself to overcome nicotine withdrawal symptoms by taking vitamin B-complex and vitamin C supplements. These will help to calm your nerves.

Hypnosis and acupuncture are the two best alternative therapies to help you stop smoking, but do not consult a practitioner unless you really want to give it up, otherwise you will waste your time and money, and do not give it up just to please others; that will not work either. If, though, you have finally decided to give up don't expect miracles. It will be a difficult road, often with many relapses, but achievable none the less.

## The weather

Changes in the weather can cause our skin to either improve or worsen. The worst time for psoriasis sufferers is said to be the autumn and at the beginning of spring. The summer can be a blessing to some or a nightmare to others, whilst the winter creates similar problems for most of us, and learning to cope with the atmospheric changes in the weather is just as important in your prevention treatment as all the other precautions you have to take to help your psoriasis.

The spring is the most likely time for allergies to become a problem. So make arrangements to strictly avoid all those foods that perhaps you risked during the winter months. Our blood tends to thicken in the winter because of the cold and through our eating more warming foods, so before spring begins you should start to eat more salads, fresh fruit and energising foods (see Chapter 8). Substitute hot drinks and soups for at least two litres per day of mineral water which will help to wash the toxins from your body.

It is better to dress warmly in the house than become too dependent on the central heating to keep you warm. Pay attention to your vitamin needs, as a change in the weather can cause viruses to be prevalent.

Just these few precautions can help to reduce the risk of increased flaking, irritation and new outbreaks of psoriasis.

During a consultation in Israel with a psoriasis sufferer from South Africa, the patient told me that his psoriasis stayed clear from the time he left Israel until the spring time in his country, and each year it returned at precisely the same time of year. On further investigation it was found that he returned home in winter and during the cold months ate a lot of spicy food. This is quite likely why his psoriasis returned when the warmer weather came.

The foods we eat during the winter months are just one of the considerations we have to be aware of. Central heating can create a very distressing amount of irritation for the sufferer, at home and in the office. As these places are lower in humidity during the winter, it means the air becomes thirstier for water, and if there is not enough water around, it will take it from your skin. A humidifier, or bowls of water placed near the central heating will help a great deal. If it is possible to keep a small window open, especially when sleeping, then do so.

Try to drink hot soups as these have a greater nutritional value than the more normally accepted hot drinks, and you must drink at least two litres of mineral water a day if you are in a centrally heated environment, if you want to reduce the flaking of your skin.

At bedtime it is better to add layers of extra blankets or wear cotton night clothes than increase the central heating.

The summer months bring them higher humidity and increased sweat gland activity helping the skin to stay moist and more comfortable. For many sufferers, though, the summer is a time of pain and torment as their skin can become very irritated. This is mainly due to toxicity of the blood and to overheating of the body, and it can be helped a great deal with the holistic approach.

Again, drink lots of mineral water, and avoid soft drinks if you possibly can. Take care of what fruit juices you choose (see Chapter 8) as they can create over-acidity. Eat mainly cooling foods, like salads, and wear cotton close to your skin which will allow your skin to breathe. Also, taking regular showers will help to control the flaking.

If your condition clears in the sun, by all means get some sun to your skin, but take the necessary precautions, and don't overexpose yourself to the sun's rays as these can be harmful in excess. Skin cancer is not something you need to deal with as well as psoriasis.

If you successfully clear your psoriasis in the summer, or it improves with some time spent in the sun, the onset of autumn can bring with it a sense of anxiety that it may return with a vengeance. This is possible, as I am sure many of you have experienced, but it can be prevented. If you follow the same guidelines as during the other months and watch the intake of your food there is no reason why the autumn should prove to be a distressing time.

Actually, some of our most distressing cries for help are received during the month of May, and just before and immediately after the Christmas period. This is probably because of a problem called Seasonal Affective Disorder, a depressive state resulting from a lack of sunlight. So, if you recognise such feelings around this time of year eat plenty of sunshine foods; that is foods that grow on trees that are fully exposed to the sun, and book a holiday.

Christmas, of course, brings with it its mix of pain and pleasure as we cope with the financial burden, the family situation, the increase in social activities and the overload of food and drink. Unfortunately, it has become so commercialised that the joy of Christmas vanishes and the emotional turmoil involved in family life really does create havoc with your health.

My advice is to take a break, perhaps departing on 26 December and returning whenever your work begins. This time is an added vacation time, so well worth considering making the best of it. It pays marvellous dividends for your skin and will help you to recover from the Christmas festivities.

# Holidays

This leads me to the next subject: planning a holiday when you are a psoriasis sufferer, and deciding where to go when you are afraid of exposing your skin. Well, actually, there are a number of interesting fun alternative holidays available to skin sufferers.

First, a short break or longer annual holiday is an absolute necessity to all of us, and should not be seen as a luxury. It provides us with a welcome diversion from daily life, gives us something to plan and look forward to and helps us to relax and unwind. The changed environment, new sights to see, new cultures to experience, tasty food to enjoy, and the fun of making new friends. All these factors help us to re-charge our batteries and restore our health.

You can take care of your skin by just a little careful planning and preparation. One solution is to take a health holiday in Israel to clear your psoriasis and then take some extra weekend breaks, another is to clear your psoriasis with the home-use UVB unit (see Chapter 2). Alternatively make a checklist of priorities in order to prevent your vacation being affected by your skin.

For example, sufferers from severe psoriasis should avoid camping, caravanning or hitchhiking holidays where there are no bath or shower facilities readily available. For those who prefer hotels, disposable sheets, pillow cases and towels can be packed as part of your luggage to avoid embarrassment. Self catering is an excellent idea as you can control more readily what you eat, and you can normally sunbathe in privacy.

If you are travelling abroad to countries where inoculations are necessary, exemption certificates are available for sufferers who experience an unpleasant reaction. We advise you to consult your doctor or a homoeopathic physician to see if there are alternative treatments available in order to avoid a reaction of your skin. Medical insurance is a must, and be sure to check the small print before your departure in case of need of special treatment whilst you are away.

During your flight drink plenty of water, and avoid alcohol, tea, coffee and citrus fruits as these will increase the dehydration process that we experience during flying, and your skin will begin to irritate and mar your holiday before it begins.

Be sure to take with you a good supply of your psoriasis

treatment in your hand luggage, wrapping it in plastic as the bottles may split due to air pressure, and suitcases can on occasion be lost. Be sure to select the correct sun tan treatment for protection and allergy factors before you leave.

Take care if you enjoy swimming, first to protect your skin by applying a natural oil like *Pharbifarm No. 2* to protect your skin from the salt if it stings you too badly, and second, remember the sea in some parts of the world can be polluted.

## Making time for yourself

Making time for some fun in your life may seem like a selfish pursuit but it is another vital ingredient to the healing process. It really does not matter whether this pursuit is intellectual and meets with the approval of your friends or just in the nature of light hearted entertainment like some of the more popular soap operas many of us are addicted to but don't like to admit it to our friends.

Blatantly planning to enjoy ourselves without including others often leaves us riddled with guilt. But why should it? We owe it to ourselves. I often visit the cinema when I need some light hearted entertainment, with popcorn in one hand and a drinks carton in the other and thoroughly enjoy myself, feeling a little like a child playing truant. I also occasionally take myself out to dinner to one of my favourite restaurants, which I can assure you took many years of confidence building, and have great fun observing others enjoying themselves. If you live alone, making life fun takes a little more practice as there is no one to jolly you along and make you laugh. Unless you work at it you can become depressed, which of course will worsen your psoriasis.

One of the most valuable tools in life for restoring and maintaining your health is a sense of humour. We are inclined to take life far too seriously for our own good. We will still experience the same trials and traumas with or without a sense of humour, and it is often our ability to laugh at ourselves that determines how we cope with these trials.

One of the most remarkable people, who I have the pleasure to say is my very special friend, is Sylvia Adler, a healer and counsellor who treats many of our patients at the Centre. The reason she is so special is her genuine ability to laugh at life and all the events it has in store for her. This ability she passes on to her patients which helps them to overcome their difficulties with more ease than more conventional health care treatments.

A wonderful piece of advice was given to one of my friends just recently by a very perceptive practitioner. It was: 'Allow some trash into your life.' He meant something frivolous, light hearted, ridiculous. It was a way of saying lighten up a little, stop paying so much attention to pursuing your life so seriously, switch off from the news headlines and read the cartoons. Being light hearted and having a little fun does not cause you to behave irresponsibly, it just means that instead of things becoming life and death situations you see the funny side. Obviously this is not going to be possible all the time as some events that happen are a matter of life and death, but many events that are testing us are not.

Very many patients tell me of their yearning to paint, write poetry, learn a language, do needlework and so on, but the time eludes them. Remember, we only have one lifetime to achieve all our ambitions, and the time goes so quickly. How many times have you looked back with regret at lost opportunities for enjoying and spoiling yourself? Well, now is the time to look forward and plan how to bring some fun into your life.

## *Peace of mind*

As well as bringing some fun into our lives, peace of mind is something we also need. Only positive thoughts and aspirations each day can help us to achieve peace within ourselves and the gift of living for today and enjoying what it brings.

We dwell on the past and worry about the future to the extent that today passes by unnoticed. This is not the recipe for peace of mind. We are so busy striving to succeed in our chosen professions, for financial security, and material possessions that we never allow our minds to rest in peace.

How many people do you know who are just not peaceful to be around? They leave you disturbed, irritated, depressed or unsettled. Those people you don't need in your life; they will not help your health. Do you have the same effect on others?

Being at peace does not mean that you have no worries or

you are not in touch with the real world. Neither does it depend on your surroundings or lifestyle. It comes from within and, like everything, has to be learnt. Meditation is a wonderful tool to begin with. You will experience a sense of peace after your therapy which will become a healthy addiction and one that is good for your health.

Another step is to become determined to think only pleasant life-enhancing thoughts. This can prove to be one of your most valuable accomplishments. I am not suggesting that you try to become a saint, but by just paying attention to the thoughts you allow into your mind, you will be surprised at the difference it makes to the way you feel, and at the improvement in your skin.

Every time a troublesome thought enters, immediately visualize a peaceful lake. Try it for yourself. Then think of something upsetting like illness or an accident and see how the picture of the lake changes in your mind. This is a sign of the effect negative thoughts have on your body, showing that they certainly don't contribute towards peace of mind. If you allow these thoughts to become more distressing and uncontrolled, the ripples on the lake will develop into a giant wave until the surface becomes completely turbulent. Now restore the peace of the lake by pushing each disturbing wave or thought one by one into the lake until the surface is once again calm and peaceful.

We have total control on our own peace of mind, it does not depend on how others make us feel, or the traffic noise, or television news, or local murders we read about in the papers. We choose what we receive, what we allow to be let in from the outside influences of life. You will be amazed how quickly you can gain peace of mind.

There are 15 sources of trouble in life that cause us all problems: selfishness; greed; uncontrolled appetites and desires; false pride; hate; intolerance; envy; bad habits (like smoking, drinking and drugs); dishonesty; living in the future or the past; miserliness; extravagance (living beyond your means); cruelty; injustice and materialism. Any one of these negative traits will prevent you from being able to achieve the total peace of mind you need to restore your health. I am sure not many of you have all of them so you could start by recognising those you do have and changing them.

The ten virtues we need to achieve peace of mind are:

honesty; truthfulness; goodness; justice; mercy; compassion; idealism; forgiveness; charity and love. Quite a tall order, but I am sure you all have some of them, the others can be gained with a little honest self-analysis and commitment.

The state of your mind affects your skin, so try to make the changes you need, as clearing your psoriasis will be the greatest reward of all.

Many of us make ourselves unhappy because we want something we cannot have. This could result from lack of money, making it impossible to buy a house, plan a holiday, have children, buy a new car. If lack of money *is* your problem, try hard not to let it be the cause of your unhappiness. Use what you have wisely and do not live beyond your means as it is so easy to do with the accessibility of credit cards. Your health is your number one priority. After that will follow happiness, success and security. Without your health and energy it is difficult to make dreams or plans become reality. Enjoy what you have now, there is no harm in desiring a better standard of living or greater luxuries as long as the desire does not become a torment that keeps you from enjoying today.

Every day something occurs that threatens our peace of mind, and we cannot ignore all the political unrest around the world, the disasters and famines reported on the news, increasing crime and violence, abuse to our children and the plight of the homeless. But we can be sure not to let them enter into our very soul and destroy our health.

One simple exercise I have practised is to keep a special word or picture in my mind, so if I feel I am being influenced by events that will disturb my mind I just switch off mentally and restore my peace by concentrating on something that fills me with pleasure. You can do this if you are in company that does not stimulate you or you discover that the people you are with are not on the same wavelength as you.

I had the privilege of meeting a young lady a few weeks ago, whose philosophy of life was something we could also benefit from. Her endless source of optimism, positive outlook and attitude never failed to amaze me. She lived alone, travelled the world by herself at the tender age of 22, had plenty of friends and it was a delight to be in her company. One day I asked her the secret of her success. She said that every day before she got out of bed she counted her blessings, reminding herself of how lucky she was. That was her formula and it certainly worked.

## *Love*

What about love, well love and peace go hand in hand as being equally important in our lives. We all need love, we were made to give and receive love in many ways. There is love associated with our children, passionate romantic love with our partners, friendship love, the love we have for the animals in our lives, the love of our parents, our love of nature and beauty.

So many of us are afraid of the emotion of love, we shy away from the word as if it is a weakness to admit to. When I ask patients how they feel about their partners they often have difficulty telling me if they love them or not. To tell someone you love them seems to imply that some sort of emotional commitment is now necessary now you have made the confession. Some will end a friendship because they realise that your feelings for them threaten to change the balance of the relationship. Others make unreasonable demands on their partners when the emotional revelation has taken place.

Love is a very complex emotion bringing with it a combination of pain and pleasure. It can make you feel very happy and fill you with fear at the same time. It certainly has an effect on our psoriasis. Don't expect that because you and your partner are in love that this relationship will make you continually happy. It takes a lot of working out, with patience and skill. Love on its own is just not enough to make a relationship last. Firstly you have to work on your personal growth and let your partner work on theirs. Loving someone does not mean they will always live up to our expectations. Love is like a very delicate flower that needs to be nourished every day and treated with care and attention. It can die so easily if it is neglected. So many of our patients suffer severely with psoriasis because of relationship problems.

# Chapter 7

# The stress factor

There is no doubt that psoriasis is influenced by our emotions. This fact can not only be confirmed by psoriasis sufferers, but by medical research and our own experience at The Alternative Centre. It makes sense, since anxiety, tension, distress, sadness, frustration and many other negative emotions do have a dramatic effect on our health. Our skin also acts as a defensive and protective agent for the mind and body in times of stress. Scratching can be seen as satisfying an unconscious need, relieving our aggressive impulses by unconsciously attacking ourselves. Most sufferers will admit that all they want to do is to tear their skin off and throw it away, and some go to extreme lengths during this thought process, causing severe self-inflicted pain, only exacerbating their suffering.

It is very important to monitor your emotions by learning what causes your skin to worsen. The physical signs are easy to detect – increasing flaking, intense irritation and increased redness, sometimes accompanied by a cracking of the skin.

One five-year-old girl, whose family had consulted us for help, had a dramatic skin reaction when she was asked how she felt about her new baby sister. Her answer was that she loved her very much but her skin reacted to this reply by visibly cracking and bleeding at the precise moment she replied to the question. Many patients will start to scratch themselves when recalling unhappy memories or when they are asked questions they don't want to answer.

Another patient experienced a severe skin reaction resulting from her inability to express the grief she felt at the loss of her dog. She was only nine years old when her mother, assuming that the dog was making her psoriasis condition worse, decided to give it away whilst the child was at school. The child, too fearful to confront her mother, had bottled up her emotions, causing an external reaction on the skin.

It is not difficult to monitor your emotions. It can be a very interesting process as you learn to overcome and control the physical reaction of your skin. Identifying the offending thought patterns is the key to success.

Negative stress factors build up in all our lives leaving us exhausted and susceptible to illness, unless we learn coping skills that can prevent them taking their toll. Such stress factors involve day-to-day events like waiting in a traffic jam, missing a train, being late for an appointment or the car not starting. Think about all the deadlines we are ruled by, hurrying from one commitment to another, arriving at work on time, or rushing to catch a plane. This is called effort-stress – a harmful and difficult habit to break, as the goals we set ourselves control our lives, and are often associated with the onset of many health conditions.

On the other side of the coin, if you are ambitious but lack the needed stimulation it is possible to become bored and lethargic, a condition which can cause as many psychological problems as uncoped-with stress, and leads to feelings of frustration and lack of self-worth in many cases. All this can bring about a worsening of psoriasis conditions as the negative energy manifests itself on the skin.

Typical sufferers of this problem are women from around the age of 30 who had given up their career to marry and have children, and the children are about to begin school. Many of these intelligent and well educated women face the frustration of not being able to get back into the mainstream of professional life.

One such case, was a woman of 35, with two school-age children who decided not to pursue a career after university because she wanted to marry. Prior to that her ambition had been to become a lecturer. Her husband was very successful so there was no need for her to contribute towards the family expenses. She was responding very well to her holistic healing programme on a physical level, but it seemed there was an underlying unresolved psychological problem that was preventing her self-healing process being completed.

Following suggestions, she started devoting time to developing her creative skills in the form of research and writing in her specialist subject area, with a view to a book and possibly a series of lecture programmes and after some weeks of this the change in her was a joy to see. By releasing her creative energy, satisfying her needs and increasing her positive stress levels, she had found the way to regain her identity, and her skin began to improve dramatically.

Another case of loss of self-esteem from too little creative stimulation was a woman of 30, with two school-aged children. This gentle, sensitive sufferer had a completely different educational background from the previous case and had left her secretarial job to get married and have children in her early twenties. There had been many problems during her married life from members of her family, and this had taken an emotional toll on her health, causing her psoriasis to become severe, and affecting her marriage emotionally and sexually.

Her skin was responding slowly to physical therapy, but there seemed to be an inner lack of the will to get well; very common with many sufferers. She had been unable to see what she had to get well for, as her life was not going to change that much if she was clear of her condition.

It was discovered that she was very creative, but like many of us did not have the confidence to put this energy into practice. Creating something with her hands was what gave her most pleasure, and some ideas were put to her for a creative programme; starting with making something as a surprise for her children. This helped her to cope with their absences whilst at school, as she had her 'secret' project to take their place during the hours they were away. It also helped to take her mind off all the family problems as her day was filled with her own activities.

Over a period of six weeks her personality changed tremendously. For the first time in many years she felt in control of her life, her skin responded well, and her family enjoyed the benefit of her renewed energy and enthusiasm. She has now developed creative skills that can help her open a new way of life, giving her a purpose and a very good reason to persevere with her healing programme.

Signs of a failure to cope with stress are irritability, constant grumbling, a tendency to flare up without real justification, a preoccupation with our health, abnormal worrying about illness, worrying about the future, dwelling on the past, and feelings of frustration or persecution. This can lead to obsessions, ritualistic behaviour, anxiety, insomnia (either all night or in the form of spasmodic sleep patterns), tearfulness, loss of energy and a permanent state of being suspicious or on guard.

All these negative factors deplete our energy, impair our immune system and make us vulnerable to disease. We are left totally unable to recharge our batteries, even after a night's sleep, a restful weekend or a relaxing holiday. Our own self-healing energy becomes completely blocked, thereby limiting our own ability to respond to any form of treatment.

Such total physical and mental exhaustion creates frustration, despair and anger as our personal and professional life becomes affected. Depression can then result making the road to recovery almost too daunting a journey to even contemplate setting out on.

Also, when we are chronically under-stressed, having no outlet for our energy, as demonstrated in the above case histories, it can also result in restlessness and depression. We pass through different experiences feeling there is no point in life, losing concentration, our approach to everyday activities becomes inefficient and we develop a repetitive way of talking.

Because positive stimulation is sadly lacking, there is a strong temptation to turn to alcohol, increased smoking, over eating, starvation diets – even the taking of drugs. We also tend to become unpleasant towards those around us, and we are liable to resent those leading more rewarding lives.

Whether over-stressed or under-stressed, the result is the same. There is a feeling of being trapped, and of desperate helplessness which becomes overwhelming when your life seems out of control. Not only do we feel trapped in our skin but also trapped by all the uncontrollable feelings and events in our lives.

Your choice of occupation can have an adverse effect on your skin. Are you competitive, overly ambitious, a workaholic? Do you travel a great deal, coping with frequent time changes, or is your occupation sedentary, monotonous and unsatisfying?

The demands of your occupation can influence the condition of your psoriasis. High stress levels are associated with lawyers, accountants, doctors, bankers, sales people and those owning their own businesses. But factory workers, shop assistants and taxi drivers are also very vulnerable. This could be the result of frustrated ambitions or sheer boredom rather than a high level of responsibility and deadline pressure.

Many high-flying executives can cope adequately with their

psoriasis (often caused by their occupational stress levels and aggravated by incorrect eating habits, irregular hours and inadequate relaxation) as long as the material rewards are there. The suffering is necessary for the rewards. The benefits gained, like an expensive house, limitless expenses, school fees for the children and the latest registration car, can seem worth suffering for.

This was the case with a lawyer who consulted us some years ago explaining that he commuted to New York from London each week to his law practice, returning home at weekends to take care of his London business and family commitments. The condition of his skin was severe and he was looking for the fastest most effective self-help therapy he could find – at any price – but was totally unwilling to make any of the changes to his lifestyle that could accommodate his skin.

He chose to stay well and truly in the 'fast' lane, regardless of the risk to his health and the severity of his psoriasis. Fortunately we were able to formulate an effective therapy, tailor-made to suit his lifestyle and needs, which he succeeded to put into practice each weekend when he returned to London, and this helped to keep his psoriasis under reasonable control.

Others, preferring to be as stress-free as possible in order to keep their skin manageable may opt for less material rewards seeing good health as their priority in life.

In our experience more and more professional men and women who are sufferers from psoriasis are ready to make drastic financial and emotional adjustments by changing their careers in order to preserve their health. This takes a great deal of courage, confidence and support from family and friends, but has been achieved time and time again.

One wonderful story shows how, when you have the will, you can find the way. After many years in the commercial world, one of our more enterprising patients came to us for help, recognizing that his inability to choose a more rewarding, emotionally satisfying career was affecting his self-healing process, and that action had to be taken as he was eager to become well.

His counselling sessions revealed that he wanted to train as a counsellor himself in order to help others, but he was unable to fund his training. Not to be defeated he decided to ask family, friends and others to sponsor his attendance for one

year at college. A good start. He successfully raised enough
money over a period of months, helped by completing a
sponsored bicycle journey throughout the country, and is now
looking forward to beginning his new way of life. Next year he
will attempt another fund-raising attempt for his second year
course.

It is important to realize the price you are paying in terms
of health and there *is* always a price. It helps to understand why
your skin is not responding as well as expected despite
choosing the right treatment for your psoriasis.

The need to change your lifestyle can be the most vital factor
in your healing programme. Believe me, there are many ways
to achieve this once you know the alternative possibilities that
are available and the practical ways to overcome some of the
very drastic changes that are associated with changing your
career. If you have the will, you will find the way and this will
help to reduce and control your own stress levels leaving you
with the energy you need to help your skin and enjoy your life.

The following case illustrates just one of the remarkable
experiences I have shared with a family who consulted me for
help in 1987, in another country, and who I have been working
with for the past three years.

The family had emigrated from America, where they had
enjoyed a good standard of living. During the first few years
in their chosen new country the father experienced an
unexpected worsening of his psoriasis and psoriatic arthritis
at the relatively young age of 35. Our consultation revealed that
they had collectively experienced a difficult economic and
emotional adjustment for which the father felt responsible.

His professional status could not be satisfactorily employed
on a full-time basis in the new land, subsequently he was
forced to accept part-time contract positions, causing financial
hardship and feelings of insecurity.

Coupled with the emotions of leaving their close family in
America, and the changes in dietary habits, the family were
all under stress. The father was very close to becoming totally
incapacitated because of the severity of his condition, which
added another dimension to their already impossible
situation.

A visit to the Dead Sea in Israel was the only immediate
solution to this problem, allowing the father to clear his
condition and cope more easily with the more practical

problems at home. After four weeks he was clear of psoriasis, and his psoriatic arthritis was greatly improved. Eating habits were adjusted, and he set off home with the promise of a new lease of life. Unfortunately a series of tragic circumstances that followed almost immediately he returned resulted in a relapse of his psoriasis, although not as severe as before.

For a few weeks he suffered, physically, emotionally and financially. In his words, in the long letter he wrote to me: 'I tried everything I could to find the answer to our problems, not wanting to admit defeat and return to America after a long nine years of effort.' He decided he had to make the decision to return to his home town in the U.S.A. to gain regular, secure employment in his professional capacity, something he had been unable to achieve in his adopted country.

Reaching this decision was a long and hard process as he was reluctant to leave his wife and two small children alone without any emotional support. The more he procrastinated the more severe his condition became. Finally, he reached the decision to go back to America for one year. He went to bed that evening with a sense of relief he had not experienced for a long time, to wake in the morning to find his skin was totally clear. A remarkable, but true story of how much the stress factors in our lives influence our psoriasis. By releasing the emotions we are able to free our minds and bodies from the burden of suffering and experience a dramatic recovery.

Another example explains how the stress of suffering from a incurable skin condition was released by a young man who had withheld all his emotions, anger, frustration and fears all of his life. After 12 years of treating his skin with many types of drug-related creams to no avail, he finally telephoned us for an appointment after being recommended by another patient who had successfully cleared his psoriasis after five months on our programme. After relaxing, the young sufferer proceeded to tell his story, explaining how he had lived with a hundred per cent coverage for a long time. He explained his feelings, the effect it had on his marriage, his professional, social and economic life. We talked for nearly four hours, and advice was given on how he could begin to help himself by adjusting his diet, learning to reduce his stress and find a more comfortable, pleasant way to treat his skin.

One week later he returned for a further consultation and told me that a miracle had happened. He had woken on the day following his initial consultation to find his skin completely clear. His wife confirmed this was the case, stating that no adjustment had yet taken place with his diet and nothing had been applied to the skin. I asked him to what he attributed this dramatic result. His answer was: 'It was the first time I have ever discussed how I felt about my condition.' He was able to see that his emotional condition was the dominating factor responsible for the severity of his skin.

By releasing all the emotions, identifying his stress and taking the necessary action to control it, with simple self-help techniques practised at home and further help on a physical and practical level, he was able to gain the quality of life he so deserved.

Enforced changes in your financial and social circumstances brought about by losing your job or the failure of a business are other stressful situations which can have an effect on your skin. All the emotions associated with such events – shame, humiliation, shock, anger, insecurity, rejection and fear for the future – can result in an outbreak for the very first time.

Taking time to adjust is important to your health and welfare and your first priority must be to take care to prevent the worsening of your condition, as this will only increase your lack of confidence and affect your ability to face future interviews.

Begin by practising the power of positive thinking. I realize this can take a lot of discipline and commitment when suffering a personal blow that affects your self-esteem. Start by convincing yourself – and you will need the undaunting support of your partner or family – that you have taken an unexpected two week vacation, and do something you previously never found time for, like gardening, reading, engaging in a hobby you always wanted to do; or take a week or two away, perhaps alone, to reassess and plan your new life.

Above all, stay active, do not allow yourself time to dwell on what has happened to you. Look at it as an opportunity to begin again, whatever your age or circumstances. Don't allow this 'interruption' in your life to make you feel inadequate or ashamed. There are millions of you all over the world in the same position.

It is a good time to assess whether you are relying too much on the latest method of treating your skin. Perhaps the time has come to begin developing your own self-help programme.

If your skin does become an added problem for you to deal with and you don't have the means to treat it in your own home, consider taking an extended vacation to the Dead Sea, in Israel, or ask your doctor to arrange in-patient treatment at your local hospital, not the ideal solution but a good temporary one which should clear your skin. Once you have cleared it can be relatively easy to learn how to stay as clear as possible.

Maintaining a purpose each day is part of your recipe for positive thinking. Scan the papers for vacancies, place your own advertisements, advertise yourself on the local radio, perhaps even set up a self-help group with others in the same situation. Contact your local employment agency, being sure to look your best at the interview, and telephone them every day without fail. Your local unemployment agency may also be able to help.

Write to companies you would like to join even if no vacancy exists, above all do not despair if the response you want does not come. Easier said than done I know, but you must have faith for the sake of your health. Keep cheerful and above all be optimistic. However long it takes, a positive attitude will bring positive results. If it has been many years since you attended an interview, then take a refresher course to brush up on your presentation skills. It will prove a worthwhile investment especially when competition for jobs is high.

For some losing a job can be a blessing in disguise, giving them the opportunity to train into something new and make the changes in their lives they always wanted but never dared to because it meant giving up a 'secure' well paid position.

Thankfully more and more of us are recognising the symptoms of over-stress and are searching for alternative ways to relieve it – an improvement on the days when to admit to an overload of stress meant you were unable to cope. Stress therapy is common sense and, as it is our responsibility to take care of our own health, not only for our own sake but for the others in our life, it must be at the top of our list of priorities.

Negatitive thoughts associated with the feelings of hope-lessness can produce chemical changes in the body. The result of a negative attitude producing negative thoughts is negative results.

A state of stress develops when these changes occur. You automatically become tense when you are projecting worry and anxiety because thinking has defeated you. The thinking process is affected, leaving you unable to make positive decisions, which in turn can leave you lacking in confidence and generally unable to cope. Even the simplest of deeds becomes too much to cope with when the body energy become depleted during this process.

On the other hand, a positive attitude will produce positive thoughts, including vivid mental scenes of success. This process will increase energy and renew enthusiasm, confidence and self-esteem. These feelings trigger chemical changes which result in a state of relaxation, thus restoring our balance.

Only you can control your thinking, and you have the ability to do so. A simple exercise of consciously changing a negative thought into a positive thought in less that one minute of it occuring can work wonders. It is just a question of re-training yourself to become aware of the dangers of allowing negative thinking and overstress to take place.

Learning to recognise and overcome stress factors getting out of control can be included in your everyday life as a matter of course. You will then be able to take immediate action to release it, and only then will you gain control over your health. The rewards are well worth the effort as you will improve your memory, your concentration, your interest in life and your energy. Perhaps you will even make the changes in your life you always wished for.

Other people and outside events do not actually cause our stress. It is our own perception and interpretation of events that determines whether or not we will produce a stressed reaction in ourselves. We cannot avoid stress altogether, as it is a necessary function in life.

It is only when it is out of control that the symptoms of stress begin to develop. It is nature's way of telling us that the body and mind need a break from the emotional and psychological factors that can destroy our health. Only then can the gradual rebuilding process of repairing and maintaining take place.

When we are not receptive to this process, illness occurs, as all stress places a strain on the central nervous system, no matter what its nature may be. If it is overworked it leads to tiredness and depletes our nervous energy, then lowers our immune system, leaving us unable to fight disease. In the case of psoriasis, it creates a worsening of the skin and can result in new lesions.

In all cases of psoriasis there is considerable tension on the nervous system and this has to be released. If we are to learn how to restore and maintain good health a relaxation programme is vital. We have to practise the art of relaxation, first by making time, and then learning the skill.

To induce a state of relaxation we have to discipline the mind to take charge of the situation, and practise the skills of letting go. Your body may be resting when you are asleep, but if your mind is disturbed, complete relaxation cannot take place.

Unfortunately there are no shortcuts to mental relaxation. Think about what little things you have allowed to build up in your mind. Are you allowing them to irritate and worry you? Are they justified, should they be there, or are you just allowing them to affect your health unnecessarily? For most of our lives we are under great tension and strain living in an atmosphere of past regret and future fears. Only by living in the here and now can you achieve peace and relaxation.

Deep relaxation techniques, and there are many interesting ones to choose from, will allow you to regenerate your mind and body, increase your self-healing energy and improve your general health and psoriasis. My experience is that psychotherapy, hypnosis, meditation, creative visualization, yoga and massage are the best therapies to choose from.

Beginning to see that we are responsible for our own illness – an excuse for the unresolved psychological problems in our lives – brings us one step nearer to achieving optimum health. This involves the metaphysical aspect of illness, meaning that symptoms can be interpreted as bodily reactions to psychological disorders. In other words, it is our subconscious that relays negative messages to the body, thus creating visible symptoms of illness, as in the case of psoriasis manifesting itself physically on the skin.

The identification of the inner problem can be difficult, as honest self-analysis is the only avenue available. Only when this is achieved can you prevent the illness returning time and time again. If the problems are left unresolved the body will continue to react.

Seeing illness as an interesting learning process, rather than a distressing situation, and communicating with your inner self, will teach you that you are the only one who is in control of your health. Only then can you make a true commitment to get well.

The formula for success is based on three words: Commitment – to improve your health; Communication – understanding your own needs; Caring – the process of self-love.

Respiratory disorders are a common complaint of psoriasis sufferers, especially those suffering with lesions above the waist. The psychological factors are fear of the contact found in relationships. Sufferers from these symptoms of the lung area are unable to accept, to give out, to gain contact with.

The skin/lungs relationship is similar, for example, in the case of asthma or eczema sufferers. When the eczema is repressed, asthma occurs, and vice versa. By holding onto the breath during the in and out process means we are unable to let go, to give of ourselves. The association of breath is that it connects us to all living form associated with contact and relationships. When our inner balance is affected because of psychological aspects, the flow of breath is interupted, and this affects our respiratory process. Resistance and fear are other associations that manifest themselves in disturbances of the heart and chest.

Psoriasis sufferers long for love, in so many cases, to make up for their feelings of lack of self-love. They want to take love, but are afraid or unable to give it, so the practice of avoidance takes over.

The liver also plays an important part in the health of psoriatics. Research carried out at King's College Hospital in London a few years ago showed that a high percentage of psoriasis sufferers had a weakness in the liver.

The liver is the largest organ in the body. It is effective in detoxification, in terms of enabling the elimination of poisons to take place via the bladder or gall bladder.

Sufferers from liver disorders suffer from loss of energy, and lose their love for many of the habits that caused the liver to become disturbed, like eating and drinking. The loss of the sex drive and potency is also a symptom.

Every symptom we experience has a psychological connotation. Arthritis, and other conditions causing a rigidity of the body structure, are related to aggression, a symptom of suppressed anger. By suppressing aggression you block your life energy. Suicidal tendencies are self-directed aggression.

Depression, another symptom of aggression, means trying to avoid responsibility associated with fear of living.

Depression is a very common factor with psoriasis sufferers, based on the continual battle of trying to overcome the condition preventing you living a normal life.

Our body is a mirror for our soul, and knowing this is a wonderful tool for healing as it allows us to get to know ourselves in a way no other can achieve. Each observation we make, we discover our innermost thoughts and feelings and can learn to analyse how they relate to our physical condition.

Symptomatic therapy has proved to be extremely effective with psoriasis sufferers, and is one of the methods taught at The Alternative Centre, as we teach sufferers how to analyse the reasons for the improvement or worsening of their skin.

Learning the gift of self-knowledge is a long-term investment and a challenge that must be undertaken with courage and commitment if you are to tread the path of self-healing. It offers the opportunity to see your illness or condition as a signal of your psychological health, and learn the valuable art of prevention therapy.

It just means we learn to see our illness as a positive step to self-development. It forces us to be more open about how we feel, to face up to acknowledging the real underlying fears and anxieties we have, which is more difficult to do than discussing the intricacies of our physical symptoms. It teaches us to look deep inside ourselves, to express what we feel, not what we think.

During many counselling sessions I have experienced many times the difficulty we have in expressing our true feelings. When a patient is asked how they feel, the answer is nearly always based on what they think. No wonder we have so many physical symptoms of illness. All our emotions are suppressed from a very early age.

Do not make the mistake of constantly looking towards others for support, understanding, and sympathy. Look inside yourself, studying your own emotions, reactions, feelings, learn to identify, analyse and solve your own health problems. Consult those who are experienced in this therapy; then you will begin to enjoy the satisfaction and contribution that can only come into your life when you understand and can take care of your own needs.

It is the buildup of the psychological and stress factors in our life that cause the problems. The smaller incidents that seemed insignificant at the time are often the ones absorbed into our mind unnoticed and without pain.

They are stored in the unconscious mind and become our own personal library. Every hurt, feeling, emotion, fear, anxiety and memory is retained, only to be released later as a physical symptom.

All of us have physical symptoms of illness, whatever age we are. Trying to establish the cause of this bodily expression of what is really going on in our mind will take patience and practice but the rewards are worth the effort, as our work in the clinic has shown.

A resistance to healing is a very common problem, and is associated psychologically with the refusal to let anyone or anything in or out. In the case of psoriasis, the skin becomes the physical body armour manifested by the mind's invisible armour which prevents the sufferer, normally a very sensitive soul, from being hurt. It acts like a protective agent and is associated with inability to let love in, stemming from the lack of self-love, the most common condition affecting mankind and responsible for so many of our difficulties in coping with life.

To receive and return love we have to lower our defence frontiers. We feel it may hurt, make us vulnerable, cause us to lose control, but love is a life-energy, a rest place for our soul and as vital to life as air and water. By resisting the expression of love, we prevent ourselves being in total harmony with mind and body. In fact we are really resisting our natural right to feel loved by resisting ourselves, not acknowledging our existence because we feel unworthy, we feel we don't deserve love, therefore we create a thick skin in an attempt to protect our vulnerability.

When we over-analyse, something we are taught from an early age of learning in the educational sense, the feeling side becomes repressed. The result is that most of our adult life is spent in conflict as we decide what we think we should do and what we feel we should do.

But underneath that protective mask lie some of the most sensitive souls I have ever met. Psoriasis sufferers have a great many problems coping with sexual activities and many shy away totally, never developing a relationship, marriage or children, whilst others successfully achieve all three.

I have talked to many sufferers about their fears of close intimate relationships and how it has affected their lives. Most long for love, and affection and have so much to offer to those willing to accept. Much of their problem lies within the own self-image projection and lack of confidence. This is also the area where lack of self-love becomes a handicap in its own right. They cannot believe that anyone would want to love them as they are so ugly because of their psoriasis.

By changing your perception about yourself, learning to recognise your most positive qualities, instead of dwelling on the more negative aspects of self-image, it is possible to enjoy a normal, happy relationship.

One young man told me that he only wished he would be able to meet someone and get married and have children but had decided it was not possible unless he married another psoriasis sufferer. Another patient said in her 30 years of marriage and four children, her husband had never seen her undressed, although he always helped her to apply her treatment to her psoriasis.

Another case was of a recently married couple where the wife, who was the sufferer, was unable to respond to her husband (who in fact was not in the least worried about the unnatractiveness of her skin), for fear he would reject her. She was very distressed, fearing her marriage would fail.

An inability to communicate to the one you love on a physical level can be as bad for your health as other more harmful practices, like excess smoking or alcohol consumption. For women who feel they have an unattractive body or skin, the devastating effect it has on their social and emotional lives is an issue on its very own. For men, where the emphasis is perhaps placed more on performance than physical attraction, another set of problems present themselves. It is no wonder that because sexual relations offer no sanctuary for disguise, exposing us in the very raw flesh, the one thing psoriasis sufferers want to avoid at all costs is an intimate physical relationship.

Many patients have told me that they feel they lost potential partners because of their condition. In some cases I suspect this is true. Sleeping beside a psoriasis sufferer who uses some of the commonly prescribed skin treatment can be unpleasant, and some sufferers have said that it actually hurts their skin physically when they make love.

There are ways to deal with these problems, which will help you to overcome some of the obstacles associated with a physical relationship. An assessment of the more positive attributes you possess is the first step. Be gentle with yourself; work consciously at replacing negative thoughts about yourself with positive ones. If you care about yourself, others will be attracted to you too. Learn to look in the mirror and see your good points, ignoring the lesions of your psoriasis. Dismiss unnecessary guilt about enjoying sex, and forget your psoriasis.

Invest in anything you feel will help you to feel better about yourself and more attractive. Spoil yourself. It may be some sensual exotic oils for the bath that do not aggravate your condition. Silk underwear is marvellously comfortable on the skin and erotic enough to be seen in the bedroom.

Romantic music, making love by candlelight or very low lights, perhaps even a glass of wine or champagne to relax you, will help you overcome your worries associated with your skin.

Buy yourself a technique manual of sexual skills, and have fun, with or without a partner, learning about the more sensitive parts of your body. Sex and lovemaking is a skill, like anything else, and has to be learnt. Invest some time into your future by removing the fear of intimacy and include making love as a necessary therapy that will benefit your health and self-confidence.

With the right partner, your feelings of shame, lack of confidence and fear of letting love in will melt away as you experience the total freedom of being able to express your innermost feelings physically and emotionally. Any protective frontiers with gradually disappear as you learn the art of trusting and self-surrender. As you begin to feel good about yourself, and your confidence and energy increase, you will discover that life without passion is like living death.

Don't hesitate to consult a specialist in this area, if you are unable to take the plunge alone. Many sufferers have fears about sex and believe that their partner will be horrified by their condition. This is natural, but many fears are in fact irrational. For example, did you know that even though your partner may sense the roughness of your skin at the beginning of making love, as it develops deeper and the blood vessels come to the surface as sexual excitement grows, and dilate, the outside surface of the skin becomes anaesthetised as the focus of the activity moves inwards? Therefore your partner will become oblivious to the condition of your skin and your skin will become less sensitive to any touch that may be uncomfortable. As a form of relaxation, sexual activity has a lot to offer.

Sylvia Adler, counsellor and healer with many years international experience in sex therapy says 'Sex as a therapy is a wonderful natural healer and is a gift to be nurtured and cherished and treated with respect. It is the ultimate form of giving, of self-surrender and of trust.

Make love with your heart and the rest will follow, but be sure that before you enter into a physical relationship that you both feel an affection and warmth for one another. This does not mean that you have to be madly in love with someone, but sex without emotion will leave you feeling empty and uncomfortable and will only deepen any negative feelings you have about yourself.

But it has to be said that most of our stress comes from trying to be something we are not. It is impossible to be successful in life unless you can feel confident and free enough to be yourself. The gift of being yourself will earn you all the love and goodwill you need to restore your health and heal your skin. All you need is the courage 'to know thyself'.

Begin by taking a good look at your body image and the effect that may be having on your mind. Looking good and feeling fit is a good way to start and will have a wonderful effect on the mind. Practise smiling and see how you feel; everyone knows the wonderful healing effect laughter has on us.

Any single deed that will increase your vitality, help you to relax, and feel good about yourself will bring about a dramatic improvement in your skin.

A great deal of psychological adjustment is required to learn to live without your condition. This has been very evident with psoriasis sufferers treated at The Alternative Centre. Even though living with psoriasis creates so many problems, losing it can be a little like bereavement, an unexplained sense of loss, especially for those who have never experienced any form of relief.

When psoriasis clears from a sufferer, they experience complex emotions. They sense they will be stepping into a new world, a world unfamiliar to the past and don't know what to expect. Fear of the unknown, of being free, stepping out of a straitjacket into a life jacket. This becomes particularly apparent when they see their skin clearing and realise this is a reality, not just another failed attempt at clearing their psoriasis. You can see the panic, the expressions of anticipation, the inner turmoil taking place as they have to decide whether to continue their therapy which will catapult them into the unknown exposing their vulnerability to what is in store without their psoriasis.

As one child of ten admitted, she was afraid that all the attention she gained from her family was something she was not sure she could live without if her skin condition cleared again. She had experienced her condition clearing some months before, for the first time since she was very young. But she discovered during its absence that the attention she had received from her father each evening as he lovingly applied her creams had vanished, leaving her feeling rejected and abandoned.

Suddenly her condition reappeared, much to her delight, and her father's attention once again was demanded. Our counselling revealed this was the objection to allowing her skin to heal once again. After a few weeks of therapy, in which she was taught how to gain all the attention she needed by giving her attention to her father in an inter-personal relationship she allowed her skin to clear and it has remained clear, much to the delight of herself and all those around her.

For adults, of course, the question of do you want to live without your psoriasis presents even more complex decisions. Especially after 30 years of suffering because our programming is more difficult to deal with. The 'invalid syndrome' is commonly known, blaming our skin for all the bad luck that comes our way, for being unable to take responsibility in our personal or professional lives. Keeping your psoriasis can seem a more attractive proposition, as at least we know what to expect from life; it is safe to live in this private world of our own, and we are experienced at living this way.

Once you have cleared your condition, you are able to see your life more clearly, to assess your needs, to make changes.

Life can only become more rewarding, have more quality and be more fun and enjoyable, if you can let go of your condition. If you don't believe me, just talk to someone who has cleared their psoriasis and you will see and hear for yourself. You can only gain what you deserve, and can inspire others like yourself to become examples of the power and control you have on your own health.

---

# Chapter 8

# The food factor

The relationship between diet, our skin and our general health is of major concern, and at The Alternative Centre we have seen a great deal of evidence that certain foods can create an adverse reaction on the skin. The national diet can be seen as a contributory factor in many countries which have a long tradition of a high intake of alcohol, meat or dairy produce. In my own case, dairy foods were the main contributor to my psoriasis. By eliminating them totally I cleared my condition, and have remained clear to date.

One particular case of ours involved a busy executive who was very distressed as his psoriasis had spread to cover his whole body, including his face and hands. He had been a sufferer from psoriasis for over 30 years, and it had become progressively worse. His wife had listened in to one of the radio helplines I was participating in, and she had contacted us for advice.

The consultation involved an in-depth analysis of her husband's lifestyle which included many business lunches as well as much travelling and never-ending social commitments. This patient was not receptive to stress therapy but he was willing to change his eating habits if there was a chance it would improve his skin.

Over a twelve week period he successfully avoided all animal products, alcohol and spices. He was so surprised to find, after suffering for most of his life, that the diet therapy worked and his skin cleared totally. He had also applied the natural *Pharbifarm* formula to his skin during this time and his words were when he visited the Centre after three months: 'I visited my dermatologist to show them my new skin and asked them why the hell had they not told me that food affects your psoriasis.'

Clinical research into the way food affects our health is conducted around the world, but very rarely is it involved in the specialist area of psoriasis. Our experience over many years has shown us that certain foods can cause the skin to irritate, itch, become inflamed and cause new outbreaks. Sadly, today many problems arise from the lack of quality of the foods we consume. Artificial fertilizers, crop spraying, and food additives threaten to be detrimental to our health and choosing the right foods for your health is as important as choosing the right partner or the right career.

The foods we choose to eat influence every aspect of our lives and yet most of us know little of the subject of nutrition and its effect on our health. If you would like to start a new way of life, studying the effect of what you eat is a good beginning.

At the Centre we are able to see the physical effect a particular food can have on the individual organs of the body using the Mora-Therapy diagnostic technique. We believe that the question of overloading on particular foods, known to affect psoriasis sufferers, does not necessarily mean in terms of quantity but in relation to the condition of the internal organs that have to cope with these foods. For example, a patient with a weak liver may suffer problems from just one or two glasses of wine, whereas someone with an efficient liver could consume more without it affecting their skin.

We are slaves to our taste buds, with addictions to chocolate, sugar, salt, caffeine, smoking and alcohol, as well as being victims of presentation, packaging, price, marketing techniques, advertising campaigns and even the psychology of colour. All these factors influence the foods we eat.

The food industry, naturally enough, is principally concerned with profits, and our health has to be our responsibility. Fortunately there is enough common-sense information available to enable us to decide and select the foods that will heal us rather than destroy us.

The choice you make must become a way of life, not just another attempt to diet. This will not work and is a waste of time and effort. It may result in a temporary improvement of your skin, bringing relief and joy, but it will quickly turn to feelings of depression if you return to your old eating habits and see your condition reassert itself.

Three particularly good books on food and health are *Complete Nutrition* by Dr Michael Sharon, *Super Foods* by

Michael Van Straten and Barbara Griggs and *Fit for Life* by Harvey and Marilyn Diamond. *Foods for Health and Healing with Remedies and Recipes* by Yogi Bhajan and *Food Combining for Health* by Doris Grant and Jean Joice are also recommended reading. (See *Further Reading* at the back of book.)

You must decide for yourself what is best for you as an individual. Your taste, income, time, lifestyle and health must be considered. Read, listen and experiment and then make your decision on what you have learnt. This way your personal choice will more easily become an enjoyable way of life.

Many natural foods are known to have healing qualities and by including them into your diet you will benefit your health and improve your skin. These foods will improve your energy and help to regenerate the cells of the body and the mind to repair themselves. They can also assist in the prevention of the ageing process and resist illness. When our energy is depleted by faulty nutrition, our immune system is lowered leaving us vulnerable to disease.

During my consultations I have experienced many cases of patients unable or reluctant to adjust their eating habits for fear of something they really enjoy being taken away from them. It has also become apparent over recent years that we just do not eat enough of the right food that produces energy. No wonder we have to put so much effort into maintaining health that it often proves too much to think about.

Marriages, relationships, businesses, your occupation, social lives and hobbies all become affected when we don't produce enough energy. The only place energy comes from is within ourselves; correct eating releases that energy for us to use creatively during our everyday lives.

Most of us are guilty of living on nervous energy, which has a severe long-term effect on the organs of the body and will affect the quality of life we achieve during later years. When you eat, what you eat, where you choose to have a meal, who you share it with, and what you talk about or think about – all can have a beneficial or detrimental effect on your health.

Eating for health and energy does not necessarily mean more time shopping and preparing foods or spending more money. Neither does it mean that everything you buy has to come from a health food store, although some specialist foods are only available at health food stores. It is good news that many of the larger food groups are aware of the growing demand for healthier, more natural foods and are making these available at reasonable prices on the supermarket shelves.

The growth in the availability of organically grown fruit and vegetables and organically fed meat is making it easier for the public to obtain better quality foods. But beware of the power of the words used to market health foods. The term 'organically grown' by itself may not mean that pesticides have definitely not been used. 'Free range' is another term associated with 'healthy' foods relating to poultry and eggs. This implies that the animals are allowed to run freely whilst they are being bred, but there is no clue as to what they are fed on. The word natural does not necessarily mean that it is safe.

Many of the natural unprocessed foods we need to improve our health can be easily obtained. All we have to do is to cut down on animal fats, increase our consumption of fresh fruit and vegetables, avoid white flour and white sugar, eliminate as many additives and chemicals from our diet as possible and, above all, enjoy the food we eat.

Counselling children and teaching them the secret of healthy eating has proved very interesting. They are much more receptive to changing their eating habits than adults, even when they have to give up some of the popular fast foods they share with their friends. As soon as they see what can be added to their diet to compensate for what they have to avoid they are ready to begin.

We encourage them to make their own list, to help educate their parents, develop their own recipes, and to keep notes on any problems or weaknesses they have problems with. More often than not it is the parents who are reluctant to make the changes in the family diet, feeling that they are depriving their children of their 'favourite' foods.

Food allergies are becoming more and more evident as a result of our bodies' intolerance to certain foods. One young patient told us that one day his skin began to turn black. A visit to his doctor showed he was allergic to grain products like bread. As soon as he eliminated the offending foods his skin returned to its normal colour and much of his psoriasis cleared.

## Milk products

Milk products, although a valuable source of calcium, have

been known for many years to be responsible for many forms of skin rashes. I have avoided dairy foods completely for over five years and a recent blood test showed no signs of a calcium problem. By balancing my eating habits and taking an effective soluble calcium supplement I am none the worse in terms of health for the lack of dairy products. The only loss I have experienced is my psoriasis, something I can definitely live with! Frequently I am asked about the dangers to health if certain foods are avoided for short-term or long-term programmes. I believe that there are always alternative ways to substitute those foods we have to avoid to gain the necessary vitamins and other necessary nutrients we need.

Many patients suffering from psoriasis have seen an improvement in their condition by cutting down on their animal fat consumption. We normally recommend that they totally avoid all dairy products for twelve weeks and then decide when they see the results whether to include them minimally on an irregular basis or to include the alternative ways to replace them. Many make permanent changes as the benefits to their psoriasis condition are realized.

We are unable to efficiently digest dairy products. Not only do they take a long time to be passed out of the body but it takes a lot of energy from the body to deal with them. The fat content tends to stick to the lining of the stomach and prevents us from utilizing all the nutrients we need from this food, and migraines, arthritis, eczema, psoriasis and many allergies have been known to be caused by dairy products.

Yellow cheeses are often made with chemical dyes known to create very unpleasant reactions for skin sufferers. Yogurt, whilst good for some, can have the same effect as milk for many of us, especially if it is flavoured and has added preservatives. It is far better to invest in a yogurt maker and make your own, preferably with goats' or sheep's milk. Although the fat content is higher the animals are not so commonly treated with the same drugs as cows.

If you find it difficult to cut out dairy foods altogether, just be aware they are known offenders to your psoriasis. Choose white cheeses, make your own yogurt, drink tea and coffee black and, for breakfast cereals, use fruit juice diluted, or make almond or sesame milk by liquidizing in a blender almonds without their skins and non-gas mineral water to the consistency you require. Dates, dried apricots or raisins, coconut and honey may be added. This healthy combination of energy foods can be used as a health drink or added to your choice of cereal. A banana, apple or any other choice of fresh fruit can also be included if you replace a meal with this drink.

Unless you suffer from allergies to certain foods and have to avoid them totally there are in fact very few forbidden foods in the health regime for psoriasis sufferers.

## Allergies

Allergies are the result of a faulty immune system. When the body is faced with an enemy in the form of a food or other substance it reacts in the same way as it does when germs and bacteria invade. It produces antibodies to destroy them. With food substances this can cause many unpleasant symptoms. Often we do not know that we are allergic to certain foods and just dismiss some of the symptoms, like migraine, constipation, tiredness, stomach pains, mood swings, depression, and hyperactivity, to name just a few, as part of the everyday problems we become used to experiencing.

Often the foods that we are attracted to – even addicted to – can be responsible for our allergic reactions. Chocolate, for example, is one of the most common foods eaten by psoriasis sufferers and an aggravating factor to the skin. It causes itching, headaches, migraine, irritable behaviour, mood swings and aggression. It can create skin rashes and spots, but is wonderful to eat, nevertheless. It is a food associated with with comfort, romance, luxury, love and is said to release a certain chemical in the brain responsible for that marvellous 'being in love' feeling.

If you discover you are allergic to this food try some of the carob chocolate alternatives which can be found in most health food stores. If it is just your sweet tooth you want to satisfy, dates, yogurt-covered fruits, or special snack sesame bars will more than adequately replace chocolate.

Research has now shown that even schizophrenia can be a disease related to allergies. In France tests carried out on sufferers linked violence and other unsocial behaviour tendencies to a reaction to coffee. Recent tests by probation officers in the north of England showed that behavioural patterns of offenders improved when their diet was changed from the processed fast foods, so popular in today's society, to a more natural way of eating.

To successfully discover if you are allergic to food, and undoubtedly many skin sufferers are, start to keep a diary of what you eat, what you combine in the same meal and at what time you eat.

A reaction on the skin can normally be detected from one to 48 hours. Monitor your skin for increased redness, itching, flaking or scaling. This way you can see if there is a problem with your diet. The only foods I have totally avoided for over five years are dairy foods and pork.

## *Vegetarianism*

This leads me to the controversial question I am often asked by patients. Should they become vegetarian? My answer is that it is something they have to decide for themselves based on the facts as we know them. I have not yet met a patient who has cleared their psoriasis because they gave up meat to become a vegetarian or vegan, which includes giving up dairy products, eggs, fish and meat.

After many years of deliberating on this subject, and attempts that resulted in failure, I must admit I have finally decided to give up eating meat. As I am unable to tolerate dairy products I guess this makes me a vegan, although I will eat fish on social occasions at home and when eating out.

What finally made me decide? Well, I have for a long time been well aware of the treatment in farming terms of the animals we eat, having talked to those closely involved. Then I began to talk to committed vegetarians about their health and their reasons, and I carefully observed their physical appearance to find visual rewards for such a dramatic change in one's eating habits.

One of the greatest adverts for becoming a vegetarian is Dr Douglas Latto who, with his equally well-known brother Dr Gordon Latto, has practised this way of life, strengthened by his love of animals, since he was very young. Dr Latto, a naturopath and gynaecologist of over 70 years of age, still travels the world and plays squash. His skin is smooth and clear and he has less lines than some half his age. He runs a busy London practice and deals with patients from all over the world.

My first meeting with him was some 15 years ago when I

visited his practice, wearing a fur coat much to his horror (something I have since given up). He recommended his own special diet, with the statement that has remained with me until this day, even though it took me fifteen years to become a vegetarian. 'How can you be healthy when you eat decomposed flesh?'

Many of my friends and family were becoming vegetarian, for moral as well as health reasons whilst I was still a prisoner of my taste buds. All attempts to convert me fell on deaf ears. I wanted to meet others that looked healthy on this regime. Not only was my health an important factor in my pending decision to give up eating animals but vanity was an important consideration too.

Most of the 'health enthusiasts', vegetarians, vegans and teetotallers I came into contact with seemed to look so unhealthy, so for a few more years I was still not able to make the change totally. A compromise was made on behalf of my health. I decided not to buy and cook meat at home, but would only eat it on social occasions in restaurants and at dinner parties.

Later, at the Centre, I came into contact with patients who had already taken the step, some during childhood, some in more recent years, and more and more facts began to emerge as one scare followed another highlighting the possible dangers to our health of eating meat. Naturally, I knew that animal protein from meat was not a healing food and can be harmful because the process of assimilation into our body takes so long, often longer than 24 hours. It begins to decay within our systems causing toxic substances to be released, putrefy and to enter our blood, overload the liver and pollute the body. Still I hesitated, but did decide to continue my search to find an agreeable alternative to meat.

I have not been an advocate of soyabean products, although many will disagree and find them very suitable for their needs, since I discovered that paint stripper was made from soya, but I would not discourage those of you from using it if you desire. I tried and tested many protein substitutes in different countries, visited vegetarian restaurants, studied ingredients of meatless diets and experimented. The main problem was the amount of time some of these preparations took and how many dairy foods are involved with meatless diets. Beans and pulses are not on my list of favourite foods, which added another problem as many of these legumes make up a staple diet for vegetarians.

We do advise patients to find an alternative for red kidney beans as they can have an adverse effect on the skin. The best advice for those of you who include these foods is to always soak them before use, boil for at least ten minutes during cooking, and be sure to mash them thoroughly before eating them. This helps the digestion process and will eliminate some of the problems associated with the consumption of these versatile, economic foods.

By changing your eating habits to improve your health, you may well experience disparaging comments from those who do not want you to seem more disciplined than they are. A word of advice for your own sanity: don't, under any circumstances, mention you are on a diet. If you do the conversation will never cease as to the why's and wherefores. A psychological battle will soon deplete your energy, the one thing you are trying so hard to avoid.

Understanding the effects the offending foods have on your skin, will qualify you to make whatever common-sense decision you choose. You make the decision to suit yourself, no-one else, and you must be selfish about it if you decide to change your eating habits. Even if you are responsible for feeding the family, you can make subtle changes either for all of you or just yourself. Don't expect the news to be received with enthusiasm, as enforced changes that affect such personal preferences as food are threatening.

## Offending foods

The suspect foods for psoriasis sufferers are excess animal fats, acids, sugars, spices, salt, and stimulants like alcohol, tea, coffee and soft drinks.

Now I will list for you more specifically the foods to avoid, then I will continue with many of the alternatives that our patients have found acceptable. To follow will be foods to introduce to your diet that will help to increase your energy and restore your health.

We recommend that all red foods are avoided. This is based on the Chinese teachings of fire on fire. As psoriasis is a red skin disease it is associated with being a fire condition in terms of a symptom. Red foods eaten by sufferers can cause the skin to become more inflamed and lead to irritation. This applies not only to the colour red but includes foods that create fire in the body like hot spices and chillies. Alcohol overheats the blood and hot drinks cause our temperature to rise.

Foods that are difficult to digest also overheat the body, as can eating certain combinations of food, like starch and protein or sugar and acid at the same meal. I am sure many of you are familiar with the irritation associated with Indian foods. The spices used for cooking are very concentrated and fiery and tend to clog the liver and kidneys. They can cause a great deal of discomfort especially if you have eaten them just before bedtime. Many sufferers from the countries associated with these foods suffer from extreme irritation because these ingredients are such an important part of their native diet.

Sugar, grapes, wine, brandy, champagne, fizzy drinks and carbonated mineral water should be avoided due to the fermentation process said to affect the liver. This discovery was made by a Dr Schafer from southern Germany some years ago, and patients we have recommended it to have experienced an improvement.

Dairy foods certainly should be avoided for at least 12 weeks, as with the other recommended foods to avoid, if you really want to improve the condition of your psoriasis. Vegetarians often overload on cheese in particular to replace meat, which could account for the fact that not many cases of psoriasis have been known to clear just from giving up eating meat.

As far as meat is concerned, beef can create an allergy response so we recommend avoiding it. Pork, without doubt, should be strictly avoided. Lamb, the Chinese say, overheats the blood, so try to do without it while you are on your detoxification programme. Sausages and patés should also be on the hit list, and fried foods congest the liver. Overloading on these foods will increase your suffering. Stock cubes for soups can have a high content of salt which can raise your blood pressure, and so should be avoided.

Some pulses can cause irritation, like the red kidney beans, but most vegetables are acceptable. However, some of our patients have reported irritation after eating potatoes. This is possibly due to the chemicals they are sprayed with, so do not eat the skins. The toxins in the skin from spraying far outweigh the benefits of fibre and the vitamins and minerals they are said to contain. Red peppers, chillies and tomatoes should be avoided.

Oranges and the skin of oranges, as in marmalade, are said to lodge in the liver and irritate the skin. (Don't worry about your vitamin C requirements as there are other safer alternative sources.) This includes the avoidance of orange juice from the stores. For the most part these tend to be very acid, do not always contain chemical-free fruit, and are often overloaded with sugar. Grape juice, grapefruit, lemon and, it goes without saying, all those canned soft drinks that are available should never become a part of your daily diet.

Many patients have reported allergies to bananas and psoriasis appearing on the face is associated with apples. This popular fruit, said to keep the doctor away, is sprayed with three times the amount of chemicals necessary, so sadly we do recommend that unless you can buy organic ones don't eat them.

Peanuts, salted, roasted or plain, addictive and tasty as they are, should be avoided by psoriasis sufferers, as should high fat content brazil nuts.

Beware of some of the fish family. Shellfish, the scavengers of the sea, salmon and smoked salmon should be substituted for other species.

Wheat and grain products have been known to aggravate the skin, but I have not yet met a sufferer who has cleared their condition by giving up bread or any other grain products. Candida albicans, a yeast infection that creates a wide range of symptoms, is related to these food substances, so if you are a victim of this problem it is likely that your skin will be affected too.

Once again, on the subject of chocolate, I would like to add that psoriasis appeared on my lower legs after eating a great deal of chocolate a few years ago whilst no other dietary habits had been changed. Beware. It is known to create problems for skin sufferers so try to avoid it if you really want to achieve success.

I am sure it goes without saying that all fast foods, like hamburgers, fried chicken, pizzas, unless the cheese and tomato has been replaced, and any other processed foods should be forgotten about.

## The alternatives

As I am sure you are relieved to see the list of foods to avoid is not that long, but I must add that avoiding just some of them and not all of them will not improve your skin as much as perhaps you are hoping. So, either make a firm commitment to embark on a 12 week de-toxification programme or don't bother to attempt it until you are absolutely sure you will remain as disciplined as you need to achieve success.

Personally I feel it takes more effort, time and money to live *with* psoriasis than it ever does to make the effort to clear it. It is just a question of re-educating your taste buds, and overcoming some of the addictive tendencies we have towards some foods.

Many of the offending foods can be substituted by attractive alternatives. Replace spices with herbs, and use celery seasoning instead of salt in popular dishes like spaghetti bolognese and any dishes you want to enhance the flavour of. Despite what I said earlier fresh tomatoes, with added water are an excellent occasional alternative to tomato purée if you cannot do without the tomato base. Purée vegetables and add parmesan cheese as an alternative to meat for pasta dishes.

Home-made yogurt is acceptable but not every day. Only use white low fat cheese, like cottage cheese, if you really have a problem cutting out dairy foods. Parmesan cheese is excellent for cooking, and on occasion the Swiss gruyère or emmenthal cheese can be used. Sesame and/or almond milk made with mineral water can be used for milk on cereals and as an alternative drink to soft drinks.

Herb teas are acceptable, but in moderation as they are very acidic. Or try very weak China, jasmine or Earl Grey tea, which are very pleasant without milk. Coffee is not a drink that helps our health as it affects the kidneys, but if you are unable to give it up, make sure you drink good quality filter or expresso, always followed by mineral water as they serve it in Europe, and limit yourself to two small cups per day. Instant coffee is acidic, and de-caffeinated coffee is more often processed with chemicals, although there are some brands that have been processed naturally. Ordinary tea, particularly the cheaper tea bags, can contain tea dust and very little of the quality leaf tea, so check carefully before purchasing it.

Some years ago I met a sufferer with 100% coverage of psoriasis. A long consultation involving every aspect of his life revealed that he drank about 30 cups of strong tea each day and had done so for many years. This was the only area in which he was overloading his system. He said he could not possibly give up his tea, so we compromised and he agree to slowly cut down to alleviate the withdrawal symptoms. His motivation was that perhaps he would at last be able to take his wife and daughter on a holiday, something he had deprived himself and them of because of his skin. One year later I met this man socially, and his psoriasis was fully cleared, and he had remained clear for a period of months after his recovery. He had succeeded in completely eliminating tea from his diet and he took brewer's yeast tablets every day. You see how simple it can be for many of us.

A soft drink now available at health stores called *Seltzer* is a very welcome change from the more common mass-marketed soft drinks. *Biotta* is the brand name for a range of mixed vegetable juices, and carrot and beetroot has proved one of the most acceptable drinks for our patients. But a word of warning, it contains lactose so if you are allergic to dairy food be sure to avoid it. *Lindavia* and *Leisure* are two excellent sources of fruit juices if you prefer to buy them than make your own. Both are available in health stores.

*Biotta* also manufacture good vegetable soups, and the *Hugli* vegetable broth is good for soup stock, in place of the more common stock cubes. This broth also makes a pleasant hot drink. Recommended spreads to replace jam and marmalade are *Awafi* date syrup, and *Chalice Foods* Carob. *Kalibu* also produce a carob powder for drinks and desserts and well as an acceptable alternative chocolate.

Don't hesitate to ask your health food store to stock your requirements. They are usually very helpful.

Oils for salad dressing should be carefully selected. Cold pressed sunflower or safflower oil is normally the best for skin sufferers, and use cider apple vinegar, never malt vinegar. Olive oil should be used sparingly. The green first pressing virgin cold pressed oil is the best quality. In the countries, like Greece, Spain and Italy, where olive oil is most commonly used there have been reports of the occurrence of dermatitis and this has been related to this product.

Unsalted butter is better than salted, and whether you use the alternatively available brands of margarines is really a question of choice. Personally, I feel that many of the oils used are suspect in terms of our health and the 'natural' dyes added can cause skin allergies.

If you are a meat eater, chicken, turkey, lamb and game seem to be the most popular with sufferers. But, please, in moderation, making sure they are fresh, free-range and organically reared. This also applies to eggs.

## Water

We have tested tap water on patients with the Mora-Therapy technique and seen for ourselves the physical effect it can have on the kidneys of sufferers. We have come to realise that not only physical problems are associated with tap water but also behavioural disturbances. Irritability in a patient is quite often associated with drinking a lot of tap water.

Evian water has been shown to improve the skin, and Volvic is the best source of water for the kidneys. It is important to alternate these regularly, otherwise you will overload on some of the minerals contained. Many patients find buying and transporting mineral water a problem, but it is worth the effort in terms of health investment, and there is probably a company that will deliver.

Water filters and water softeners have proved very popular as an alternative to consuming the pollutants that come from drinking water directly from the tap. But there is a specific process that must be part of the water filtering technique called reverse osmosis. It would be worth your while considering having a good quality water purifier installed in your house.

I advise you to use either bottled or filtered water for cooking and for drinking. Pure water is a necessity not a luxury and must be included in your weekly shopping for the sake of your health.

## Alcohol

It is equally important to know the potential liver damaging effects of prolonged excessive alcohol consumption as many psoriasis sufferers have problems with their livers. Alcohol is an 'empty' calorie food and contributes towards raised fat levels in the blood and to poor blood sugar control.

There is a tendency for psoriasis sufferers to use alcohol as a consolation, and run the risk of drinking too much for their health. This can have an unpleasant effect on the skin by increasing the itching and flaking, so it is important to be aware that drinking can have an adverse effect on your self-healing programme. It does not mean you have to become teetotal, but knowing the facts will enable you to adjust your habits to suit your needs.

Alcohol is a toxic substance which in excess depletes your body of essential nutrients. These include vitamin K, zinc, magnesium, potassium, vitamin C and some of the B vitamins. It also affects the liver in that it renders it unable to effectively deal with the elimination of waste, and it affects its ability to metabolize glucose. It can contribute towards overweight, prostate problems in men, thrombosis, sterility and a wide range of psychological and behavioural problems, like anxiety, panic attacks, depression, and violence.

If you are partial to a glass of wine, try to drink only white. One of the nicest alternatives is to try a combination of wine and carbonated or still mineral water, known as a spritzer. There are plenty of non-alcoholic beers available as well as some excellent non-alcoholic wines. Alternatively be sure always to drink mineral water after each glass of wine, this not only helps to prevent irritation but will help to eliminate the rather unpleasant after-effects associated with alcohol.

## Coffee and tea

The damage coffee and tea can cause with excess consumption is something you should be aware of. Tea, of course, could be classed as an epidemic amongst the British. Both these drinks are stimulants because of their caffeine content. It gives you that necessary 'lift' to get you going, especially in the morning, but its effect is only temporary, and it depletes your energy more rapidly than we realize.

Caffeine on an empty stomach is said to cause an excess secretion of stomach acid which encourages ulcers. As it raises blood pressure it can contribute towards heart attacks, and it has also been implicated in the formation of kidney stones, and in the incidence of certain cancers. Tea contains tannin, which badly affects the secretion of digestive enzymes, and the alkaloid theophylline, which is an irritant to the nervous system and is much more potent than caffeine.

As with alcohol, if you want to drink tea or coffee, drink it very diluted, and follow it with water. Herb teas are really worthwhile contemplating as alternatives.

# Sugar

Date syrup, maple syrup and honey are excellent alternatives to white sugars, whether for sweetening drinks or for cooking. Keeping our blood sugar at the correct balance is the function of a complicated hormonal process which becomes over-worked if we consume far in excess of our needs. An increase in protein can help you overcome your need for sugar, this helps the adrenal glands and pancreas stabilize the sugar level. This can come from grains, legumes and seeds which provide a combination of protein and starch.

# Frequency of meals

We are conditioned from childhood to eat at certain times – usually to the routine of three meals a day – but a more suitable pattern is to eat little and often. The established habit is hard to break, but it can be achieved without losing the social side of eating together. If you eat little and often during the day, to maintain your energy, it just means you will eat less in a social or family situation. Also practise eating when you are actually hungry and not just because of obligation, for comfort or to alleviate boredom. This not only gives your digestion a rest but will allow you to monitor your needs more accurately.

# Foods for optimum health

My recommendation for regaining optimum health is to select your foods in terms of their energy content. Only eat what will assist you to release your own energy, this way you can enhance your holistic health programme and help to clear your skin.

Fruit for breakfast is an ideal way to start the day, taking care to avoid the acid and red fruits, like oranges, grapefruit, limes, raspberries, strawberries and red currants. Goats' or sheep's milk yogurt can be added if you have a problem giving up dairy foods, but not every day because you will overload your system, and become impatient if the results you are looking for do not come. Alternatively, make your own home made fruit drink. If you still feel hungry wholewheat toast with honey is acceptable.

Melon is one of the best fruits to start the day with, as it is an excellent cleanser of the liver, and the seeds are high in vitamin E. It is assimilated and passes through the body in about 20-30 minutes, so is not demanding on digestive energy. Eating one fruit at a meal is actually better than a selection as the combination of different enzymes can affect your digestion process. Eat any fruit at least 30 minutes before you eat other solid food.

Salads with jacket potatoes (but don't eat the skin), tuna fish, sardines, eggs, feta or cottage cheese, almonds, sesame seeds, avocado (a wonderful food without cholesterol for increasing energy), perhaps pulses, pasta and meat (if you want it) are some of the ingredients you can combine. Be sure to add watercress, which contains calcium and helps blood pressure. Celery is beneficial for women as it helps to alleviate water retention associated with PMT and is beneficial to the nervous system. Garlic, nature's antibiotic (called Russian penicillin) is another good ingredient for salads and other dishes.

If you enjoy pasta, look for semolina or durum wheat pasta – wholewheat if you prefer (I know it is healthier, but personally I find it a little too heavy to eat.) Wild, Mexican and basmati rice combines very well with vegetable combinations.

Pineapple aids the assimilation of protein if eaten before a meal and can help with digestion problems. It also aids the body in eliminating waste through urination by assisting the liver and kidneys. Dates, a sunshine food, are a natural laxative and an instant source of energy. Parsley is also a natural diuretic, rich in minerals that help the blood, cleanse the kidneys and help to balance calcium. Eaten after garlic, it helps eliminate the smell from the breath.

Lecithin in liquid, granule or tablet form is known as a brain food. It helps the nervous energy, improves memory and helps skin conditions. It can be added to soups and health drinks.

Almonds are a good source of potassium, calcium and phosphorus and are another energizing food, especially for children and babies as it can be made into a milk or almond butter by mixing it with lemon juice.

Coconut, raw, dried or milk, is a food not so commonly associated with our diet but is easily digested and contains all the amino acids that provide protein plus vitamins and minerals. Added to rice, in a health drink, or in any recipe, it is delicious, but don't use it too often as it can cause you to put on weight.

Molasses is the raw product from sugar cane and is rich in minerals and trace elements. It is an alkali-forming food and excellent for arthritis and general health.

I have heard reports from patients with thinning of the hair due to scalp psoriasis that taking one tablespoon of molasses each day in hot water, and drinking it through a straw (immediately cleaning your teeth afterwards as it can stain and damage your teeth) for six months has improved the growth of their hair.

I must ask you to note that if you are considering becoming vegan or vegetarian, be sure to have a regular check-up to ascertain that you are not creating any nutritional deficiencies whilst you are in the learning process.

As important as choosing the right foods is to keep your body clean on the inside with a diet of high water content foods – 80% of your diet in the form of fruit and vegetables. This will help your body detoxify daily.

A way of eating which has proved to be very effective is the Hay System, named after an American doctor, William Howard Hay early this century. It concerns itself with food combinations, and the basic idea is to avoid mixing protein foods with starches or sugars in the same meal.

The easy way to do it is to write a list of the foods you normally eat in a week, then divide them into starch foods and protein foods and take care not to eat them within four hours of each other. The same applies to acid and sugar foods.

There are foods that *can* be combined with starch and protein. These are herbs, seeds, like sesame, sprouted seeds, like alfalfa, sunflower, sesame or olive oil, cream, butter, egg-yolks, all vegetables, and all nuts except peanuts.

Finally the psychological reasons for so many digestive orders have to be considered before you begin your new way of eating.

It is important to understand what is going on in your mind that is causing you to have a problem with the foods you consume. This inner conflict affects psoriasis sufferers since the tension factor is always high as they battle with the condition.

Think about the foods you cannot tolerate, what is it in your mind that you cannot tolerate. Perhaps it is just being a psoriasis sufferer or something from way back in your childhood. Whatever it is it has to be dealt with, either alone or with the help of professionals. Ulcers are graphically a symptom of us digesting ourselves as the walls of the stomach are attacked. By becoming more aware of our thought processes and how they affect our digestion we are able to help ourselves by analysing why we are in conflict with ourselves, what it is we are looking for – love, security, dependence. Are we repressing our aggressive tendencies, or eating our hearts out?

During our lifetime many of these mixed emotions occur, all we have to be aware of is what is causing them and how to solve them. Are we guilty of finding faults with ourselves or others, are we living in fear? Do we overeat because we fear hunger or perhaps we feel we are not getting enough of the things we deserve? Constipation is also a common problem with psoriasis sufferers and is associated with the reluctance to let go.

If you study and understand the holistic way of healing that includes this alternative eating plan, you will appreciate that these changes, daunting as they may seem in the beginning, really will allow you to change your way of life and heal your skin.

A long healthy life is what most of us are aiming for and it does not just happen: we have to plan it with the same precision as you may well plan your career. Every morsel you eat, every liquid that passes your lips, every thought process you allow to manifest in your mind has a positive or negative effect on your life.

Choose, natural, unprocessed foods, use only wholegrain breads, brown flour, brown sugar, as many fruits and vegetables as you like, cut down on animal fats, acids, dairy foods, and sugar. Carefully combine the foods in order to increase your natural vitality, maintain your energy, and to improve your digestion and elimination processes, and enjoy the art of alternative eating for health.

I have seen many cases of an 'improvement' in general health of psoriasis clearing by adopting this new common-sense approach to eating. If you really want to help to clear your psoriasis, then start now and make it a fun experience.

# Chapter 9

# Do you have a child with psoriasis?

Many more babies are born with eczema than psoriasis. Nevertheless psoriasis can occur in children at an early age. Research carried out in France has shown cases of pustular psoriasis occurring in infants as early as three months old. In some cases these conditions are severe, and by the time the child reaches puberty their condition resembles that of an adult.

In a recent study 45 per cent of psoriasis cases started before the age of 16. The most common form that affects children is *psoriasis vulgaris*. There are rare occasions when a newly born baby will have psoriasis-like lesions. The condition often manifests itself on the scalp first and then proceeds to the body. Similar factors as in adults cause the onset of psoriasis in children. Infections, like tonsillitis or stress factors at home, family or school, and the worsening of the condition can be provoked by the use of systemic drugs that are intended for adults.

PUVA is rarely recommended for the treatment of psoriasis in children. Treating children with orthodox medical prescribed treatments has not proved very successful as parents are more concerned about the possible side-effects.

In many cases of childhood psoriasis there are hereditary factors involved. Sometimes, cases of congenital *psoriasis universalis* is diagnosed as *Ichthyosiform dermatosis*. To identify your child's skin condition look for irregular-shaped slightly raised skin, covered with scaly patches. The elbows and knees are especially affected, and the scalp condition could be easily mistaken for dandruff and made worse by dandruff shampoos. Look also for pitted or ridged nails. It is said that there is no itching with psoriasis, but experience shows that washing powders, detergents and certain foods do cause irritation.

The soreness of psoriasis makes close contact with your child very difficult and can seem like a wedge between you. Your child may react with tears, temper tantrums, appear irritable and restless and cause you a great deal of concern, frustration and sleepless nights. If neither of the parents are sufferers themselves, and are unable to experience what the child is feeling, it becomes an even more difficult problem to deal with.

The first thing to do is to read everything you can on the subject to enable you to understand the physical condition of the disease. Don't despair if the words 'cure' or 'clear' are not referred to in medical books on psoriasis. You *can* clear your child's psoriasis, just the same as clearing an adult's. It's just a question of knowing how. The most valuable gift you can offer your child, as well as love, is to allow him or her to learn how to manage the condition, at however young an age. I don't mean manage in medical terms by applying the latest prescription, but rather by encouraging an understanding of the holistic way to restoring health. Your child will be growing up in a generation which has a greater awareness of the natural, alternative ways to heal, and of the value of preventative medicine. Such therapies will hopefully be integrated with orthodox medical practices and thereby offer a more comprehensive approach to health.

Guilt is not an uncommon emotion for the parents of a child who has become a skin sufferer, especially if one of you is a sufferer also. Remember, it is not your fault, it is just something that has occurred within your family and can be dealt with intelligently and rationally. One man, in his early fifties, receives money every month from his mother for his psoriasis treatment. His wife says she was sworn to secrecy never to tell her husband that his mother has also been a sufferer for most of her life, but had decided to remain in the 'closet'. By paying for his treatment she is able to alleviate some of the guilt she feels.

The natural tendency you will feel to spoil, and over-compensate your child can prove fatal for the family as they will soon learn to become self-centred and manipulative. The very fine balance between too much and too little attention is going to become quite difficult to achieve, but you can learn. You will also learn to recognise the symptoms of the invalid syndrome, the behavioural problems, the temper tantrums. It doesn't take long once you become aware.

Be sure to explain to your child very carefully exactly what psoriasis is in physical terms, and then explain how the psychological aspects of our lives can affect our skin. The next step is related to all the ways they can help themselves.

Children brought up with common sense, honesty and tender loving care are such a pleasure to deal with. They have no pre-conceptions, no elements of mistrust, no sides, they do not dismiss therapies before they have tried them. Some of our fastest healing has taken place with children. If you don't feel equipped to handle the situation or have not gained enough knowledge to pass on to your child, consider seeking advice from a specialist clinic. At our Centre we show parents and children how to tackle the problem in a fun and pleasant way, which can avoid hospital visits and all the traumas they entail, and the drug-related creams.

One of the most important things for your child to understand is that he or she is not alone, like so many assume. One little boy of eight whose family consulted us recently told us he was the only boy in his school with psoriasis. His suffering was made even more acute as he had severe lesions on his face, and things were made yet worse by the emotional upheaval of his parents' recent separation. We put him in touch with a young patient of 10 as a pen pal, because up to then he had never had any contact with another sufferer.

Even though of little real consolation, it is worth getting the child to appreciate that there are many very much worse off. This can help them to grow up with the strength and resilience to cope with life, despite their handicap. It is how they feel about themselves that counts. Confidence in handling their own problems from an early age results in the child becoming a healthy and well-balanced adult.

Teach the child that the most valued thing about a person is not their physical appearance, but what is in their head. It is not him that the other children are rejecting, but his skin condition.

## Finding the right treatment

It is important, of course, to get the correct diagnosis before treating the condition. Above all, take extra care not to show anxiety or frustration if the treatment you have chosen does not improve the condition. Your child cannot respond to treatment to make *you* feel better. Different treatments suit different people.

One of the most difficult things to do is to stop your child scratching when the skin itches. One teacher of a 10 year old skin sufferer reported: 'The more I tell her to stop scratching the more she does it.' Keep finger nails short, and when the skin itches suggest gentle rubbing rather than harmful scratching which will break the skin and cause it to become infectious. Remember it is always more difficult for your child not to scratch when the skin itches than for you to watch them. Distracting their attention with hobbies and games is more effective than threats or nagging.

One of the classic family situations is when the child feels inadequate because they are unable to respond to their parents' well-intentioned efforts to banish this distressing condition – efforts that become part of every day, affecting the financial, emotional and psychological aspects of family life. In such cases the child can become more and more withdrawn, alone, and desperate for someone to understand how they are feeling.

One caring mother, whose son had suffered from psoriasis since he was a small child, made it her sole purpose in life to find a cure for him. With every new treatment she discovered, a twice-daily inspection was carried out to check for improvements or new outbreaks. Her impatience for immediate results, and every disappointment they experienced (often because treatments had not been used for long enough), resulted in a personal feeling of failure experienced by her son. He was unable to clear his psoriasis and please his mother.

Her good intention of wanting to see him free of suffering had become an obsession, and greatly contributed towards the emotional distress, and lack of confidence he was still experiencing at the age of 25. All this, plus having his attention continually drawn to his condition, which he was longing to ignore, caused his psoriasis to become more stubborn than ever. This made it even more difficult for him to respond to treatment. Careful counselling eventually made her realize the error of her ways, and she subsequently relaxed her impatient approach to clearing her son's condition.

From a very early age your child will be able to understand

many spoken words, even though they can themselves only utter the odd one. So, take care not to make the common mistake of discussing the condition of their psoriasis, thinking that your child cannot understand what you are saying. Psoriasis sufferers are particularly sensitive souls at whatever age.

It is, of course, important to take maximum care when looking after your child's skin. For babies it is possible to buy an all-in-one suit in cotton to help prevent irritation. Also, allow them to run around without clothes on so that the air can circulate their bodies. This is especially helpful when they are going to bed.

Sleep is another important factor to your child's health. Children burn up a tremendous amount of energy, as they seldom sit and relax, so they need at least twelve hours sleep during those growing years. The condition of psoriasis causes the sufferer to lose valuable heat and energy and can only be restored when the body heals itself in the state of sleep.

Some parents are reluctant to let their children sleep during the day in case they don't sleep at night. Relaxation therapy and a gentle herbal tea will help with these problems. You will notice a remarkable improvement in the skin if your child has enough quality sleep. A flare-up in the condition of their psoriasis, bad temper, irritability, or crying are tell-tale signs of insufficient sleep.

The skin will show signs of being more 'angry' and red, and flaking is normally more prevalent when they are tired. There is a tendency to scratch more often, and with greater intensity. If you check the skin after a good night's sleep, you will see a change of colour – more pink in appearance, instead of red, and the surface feels smoother to the touch. Allow them to sleep as long as they want. Nature has a way of taking care of our needs. They will soon be subject to deadlines for waking when school starts.

## *Monitor your child's emotions*

Monitoring your child's emotions is very important in identifying what causes a reaction in their psoriasis. We must remind ourselves what it felt like to be a child in a world of adults. Children do not have the confidence to express how they feel, and because they don't communicate with us we tend to assume that they are either not suffering or are able to cope. Having a skin condition makes them feel even more isolated, especially if they don't know anyone else with the same problem. Suppressing their emotions is, without doubt, one of the most harmful behavioural patterns for them to learn. It can easily occur as parents don't always have, or make, the time to encourage them to learn the art of expression. Many parents are unable to express their own feelings, let alone become good teachers. Learning to communicate their feelings to you without fear of reprisal, ridicule, or being misunderstood, is one of the greatest gifts you can teach them and will help them to relieve their psoriasis as well as grow up into healthy, happy, successful human beings.

One of the ways to monitor emotions is to take note of when your child is scratching or nibbling the skin. You can then ask them if it is as a result of something they are thinking about or something they have eaten. It is a good idea to suggest to them that they keep a little notebook or diary to monitor their own responses, and to keep a list of the offending thoughts and foods. Most children I have dealt with have enjoyed this exercise and taken to it willingly. Teaching them to see their condition as an interesting subject and not a destructive one will prepare them very well for coping with psoriasis as an adult. Don't do this for them if they are old enough to take responsibility themselves. On the subject of food, use the guidelines in the food factors chapter.

## Change of diet

It will prove more difficult to change their diet if they are used to the more normal foods the children of today seem to eat. But you should find that, by gaining their co-operation which will come from your careful explanation on why they have to avoid certain foods and why they make psoriasis worse, you will encourage them to adopt a regime of healthy eating. Let them make their own adjustments in their own time. Even encourage them to prepare their own food, and make up their own recipes. Don't worry about the mess they may make, a happier child in the house is worth a little more work. Above all, do not reproach them if you see them eating foods that aggravate their skin, just turn a deaf ear to their complaints when they experience a reaction and don't let them cajole you into trying yet another treatment, and spend yet more money in the quest for an easier, quicker way for them to improve their skin. Dietary adjustments work for most sufferers, and some results should be noticeable after 12 weeks. They may not fully clear their psoriasis in 12 weeks, since there may be many other complex emotional issues involved. Remember how clever they can be at gaining attention, they may not want to lose their condition or show signs of improvement fearing the loss of love and caring. Some cannot visualize living without it.

Refined sugar is something you must make a determined effort to get your child to give up. Be patient, and gradually introduce the recommended substitutes. Start buying the natural foods like honey, carob chocolate, etc. Don't feel you are depriving your child because he or she is not having what other children have.

Depriving children of a chance to heal their skin is even more of a sin, but don't scold them if they decide to follow in the footsteps of other children. Just let them be, they will find their own way in their own time of re-adjusting their diet. As a parent it is your responsibility to show them the right way to help their skin. Just offer the information, or write it down and present it. They have the right to make their decision of what to do with that information. Tell them not to discount it until they have tried it.

I know it's easier said than done, especially for mothers to hand the responsibility of their child's health back to them, but it can be done gently, slowly and gradually, with you persuading and selling them the idea, not telling or dictating. I have seen the faces of parents in consultations when their child is present. Just the sheer fact that the child sufferer is writing down all the foods they cannot eat and all the foods they are encouraged to eat. The parents are often quite bewildered by the willingness and interest their offspring shows in self-help.

Certain foods are vital for the growth of children and it's important to know which ones will help them to become strong and healthy. Let's start with babies. First, the way you feed and what you feed your child with will build their foundation in terms of physical and psychological health, so your choices are very important – even more so if psoriasis is presenting a problem.

Likes, dislikes, habits and attitude towards food and eating develop at a very early age. If you possibly can, breastfeeding is advised, as this is what nature has intended and not only does it help strengthen your baby's immune system but also helps the bonding process. It also provides all the necessary nutrients, is pure and easier to digest.

Almond milk and walnut milk is recommended for children. Start with just a few teaspoons per day, but only after above three months old. Sesame or almond oil, only three drops a day, will help to digest nut milks, and will benefit the skin.

As soon as teething begins the child can begin to handle more solid foods, but be sure to mash or blend. Start with fruits, but avoid the ones known to aggravate psoriasis. Introduce new food slowly, perhaps trying one food for a few days to check for any allergic reactions. Watch for unexplained changes in behaviour like continual crying, extra sleepiness or inability to sleep, and rashes on the skin.

Baked apples and bananas, mashed, are a good healthy start, but avoid including the skins from the apples as a preventative measure against any preservatives the apples may have been sprayed with. Try if possible to find organic fruit. Later you can introduce other fruits known to be especially good for children with psoriasis – advocados, peaches and pears. As for vegetables, carrots are an excellent starter. But introduce vegetables slowly and only one vegetable at a time, as with fruit, to avoid overloading the delicate digestive system of your child. A few drops of cold-pressed sunflower oil added to the puréed vegetable will help the assimilation process.

Almonds and walnuts can be made into nut butter. Children's digestive systems cannot cope with whole grains or nuts so be sure, even with rice or grains, to mash or purée them.

Yogurt and cottage cheese can be digested by young children, but hard protein is more different. It is recommended that they should not eat hard cheese before three years old. Certainly if you have a skin condition it is better to avoid it altogether. Try goats' or sheep's yogurt in preference to the ones made with cows' milk, but use products sparingly as they have a higher fat content.

Once your child is old enough to communicate when they are hungry, teach them to listen to their needs, by allowing them to eat when they are hungry and not compelling them to eat when you decide. I have seen this process work very well in a family with a small boy in Switzerland. His mother told me, on one of my babysitting assignments: 'When Dino goes to the fridge door it means he's hungry, just take a piece of fruit, or whatever he reaches for, and let him have it.' As Dino and I did not speak the same language this seemed an ideal solution to the problem of communication. Only later, after many subsequent visits, did I discover that this was a normal part of the daily routine of eating practised by this healthy contented two-year-old. He was not expected to join the family for dinner, although now he joins them for every meal and has done so since the age of four, at his own discretion. Observing this rather unusual procedure in child upbringing, I soon became convinced that it could be carried out with the minimum of convenience and fuss and work well for both the child and parents. I am convinced that so many eating disorders that occur later in life are as a result of being expected to eat when we are not hungry as children, being overfed, and eating foods we really don't have a taste for but feel compelled to eat as they have been prepared for the whole family.

We feed babies when they make it known to us that they are hungry, which is normally when they cry. So, they are used to eating when they are hungry, which may be five to six times a day or more – in other words, they eat little but often. As soon as they are able to sit in a seat at the table they are normally expected to eat when we eat, and we almost forbid them to be hungry in between our regulated mealtimes, in case it spoils their appetite.

This only introduces the habit of overeating at the 'allowed' three mealtimes a day, and sets a pattern of feeling we are not allowed to show we may be hungry in between times of meals. Does this sound familiar? If it does, see how you can adjust things. You will probably find you are serving less foods at mealtimes and your children are happier and healthier.

Be sure to make accurate assessments concerning your child's eating habits and needs. Very young children at around one and two use a lot of energy but cannot digest a great deal of foods at regular mealtimes, so it's advisable to consider giving them something to eat about every two hours. Older children normally are happy being fed on a less regular basis.

Adult psoriasis sufferers have a common problem with the digestive process. So, by teaching your child to relax, feel peaceful and comfortable and eating their food with care and attention and with respect for their body, you will prevent them from suffering unnecessarily later in life. Explain how the body works, how it assimilates the foods, and how to prevent elimination problems.

If the pain of teething is causing eating problems, rice bran syrup, as a supplement available in health stores, is a good source of nutrients and will help to prevent appetite loss. Celery juice is good for both of you as it helps to soothe the nerves. Serve it as a vegetable soup or a hot drink if it is unacceptable cold. Carrots are good for chewing, after being well scrubbed, for teething and a little clove oil applied to the gums helps to numb the pain.

Don't encourage them to eat hot, spicy foods as this is certainly not recommended in cases of psoriasis. Remember, if you are tasting food before giving it to them, your taste buds are more cultivated and the food may be too strong. Let them be the judge of the blandness or flavour.

Just the same guidelines apply as to your health in that you must try to avoid chemically sprayed foodstuffs, and tinned and processed foods. We also recommend highly that you take extra care in reading labels for offending additives and preservatives. Any mother with a hyperactive child will tell you of the effects they can have on such a child's behaviour.

One family reported that their son, from less than one year until nearly five, suffered from hyperactivity in the most extreme way, which worsened his behaviour almost to the point of being totally out of control. Eventually the offending allergens were discovered, allowing the distraught mother to abolish all those foods containing additives that were damaging her child's health. I witnessed the effects of the offending foods on this otherwise normally behaved, lovable boy over those years and it was very distressing.

So, don't underestimate the effect these additives can have on your children, even if the symptoms are not so noticeable as in this case. Our advice is that if there are additives in a product, put it back on the shelf. An excellent book to help is *E for Additives* by Maurice Hanssen and Jill Marsden (Thorsons, 1987).

Try not to introduce your children to junk foods. So many of the children I see only seem to want to eat junk foods. In the mass-market food chains, with their many years of successful marketing, every effort is made to encourage families to treat their children. If your child has a skin condition, the fat content of most of these popular foods is just not conducive to their psoriasis, and once they are indulged, it can so easily become a habit that is hard to break.

Try to avoid sugar and salt in their diet, they both have addictive factors and can safely be substituted with far healthier alternatives. Children also need lots of fluid, but certainly not in the form of the popular colas. Try to introduce the benefits of natural still mineral waters at an early age. You can add a little fruit juice to it as long as you avoid the ones that will aggravate their skin, like orange, grapefruit and lemon juice. On no account introduce them to squashes or sweetened water by means of adding sugar, you will only awaken the sweet tooth syndrome. Try to teach them to drink at least half an hour after eating. It will help their digestion.

Give your children a chance to grow up in good health by laying the foundations as early as you can. You owe them the right to good health. Don't attempt to introduce vitamin or mineral supplements before the age of five. If your child is being fed healthily there will be no need. An imbalance can be created in the body by giving unsuitable supplements to your child, and if they are thought necessary professional advice should be sought.

How do you prepare and teach your child to cope with psoriasis as they get older? The answer is with tender loving care, patience and understanding. All manner of emotional and social pressures will have to be overcome during their development years if your child is going to emerge relatively unscathed from his experience.

If children feel loved and secure in the family unit, it will provide them with the confidence needed to face the outside world. Encourage them to make friends, and inform them about the condition so that they can answer any questions that will undoubtedly arise. Be sure that the parents of the children your child is mixing with understand what psoriasis is and that it is not catching.

It is surprising how many people have not heard of this very common skin complaint. Children are never too young to be taught to be aware of the needs of others. This can be an invaluable healing tool in their therapy and to help them to replace the attention they may be afraid they will lose if their skin heals.

## *Physical contact*

Children with blemished skin, as as with any other handicaps, need compliments, to be hugged and shown a great deal of love. It's surprising how our busy days don't always leave us with the time and energy to carry out such little but very necessary deeds. The physical contact is essential since it is all so easy to allow a sore skin to create a barrier between you. A baby with a sore skin often receives physical contact many times a day until it is able to move unaided. After this physical contact decreases since the child has now become more independent and no longer needs to be picked up.

As children grow older they receive less and less physical contact from their parents and relatives to the point where it becomes almost non-existent. The warmth and security associated with a hug from someone close is something we all need. It's part of life energy and love, and essential to our health and well-being. Children and adults with a handicap are even more in need as they live with their own personal feelings of isolation and rejection.

## *School*

Coping at school is another big step for your child. This period can be particularly traumatic if they are suffering from something as visibly unpleasant looking as psoriasis. One of the first lessons for them to learn is how to become more confident in their relationships with other children and teachers. Your encouragement and support and patience is vital. I was a psoriasis sufferer at school and can still remember how shy, embarrassed and lacking in confidence I was, and this did not help my academic progress. One point I feel is important to mention is that I have found many children with psoriasis have been able to deal with the creative side of school subjects, with some excelling in this area, rather than the other subjects involved in the school curriculum. This has also been evident in adult sufferers looking back on their schooldays.

It has often helped for parents to recognize and encourage their child to develop creatively, and it can relieve some of the pressure they have experienced at being unable to keep up with other children, which in turn, of course, relieves some of the emotional distress that inevitably affects their skins.

It is important for you to make an appointment with your child's teacher to be sure they understand the condition and what it involves in terms of physical and emotional distress to the child. One mother reported that her ten year old's teacher said she was convinced her child was scratching on purpose to annoy the teacher, as every time she told this distressed young girl, who was the only one in the class to suffer with a skin condition, to stop scratching she did it even more obviously. To those of us experienced in all the influences involving skin conditions, the emotional distress this child was subject to every time the teacher drew the attention of the whole class to her suffering caused her skin to irritate even more.

Physical training instructors and swimming coaches should also be informed, as sports clothing does not conceal the skin and your child will be unwilling to participate in any sporting activities if they are unsure of the reaction of the other children. Any treatments that have to be carried out during school time should be clearly understood by the teacher as well as any necessary precautions that have to be taken, or dietary adjustments.

Your child will be very embarrassed if the flaking shows because you have not informed the teacher about the necessary treatment that has to be applied to keep this at bay. A written guideline from you will be a great help to the teaching staff. This should include instructions for treatment, whether your child needs help with application of it, how best to handle scratching, and necessary food precautions. Consider the possibility of packed lunches if the school meals are not in accordance with your child's guidelines. Don't hesitate to enlist the support and co-operation of the head of the school as they are normally sympathetic. With 4 per cent of the population under 12 years of age suffering from eczema, children with skin problems will not be an alien problem for them to deal with. Many parents I have spoken to have voiced their hesitation in enlisting the co-operation of teachers, but you owe it to your child. Remember those most important growing years are spent in the care of strangers at school, so don't deny them the best care during this important time. It will benefit your child for the rest of their life.

Be careful not to make the mistake of one anxious mother. She decided it would be best for her son's welfare if she enlisted the help of the headmaster of the school which he had been attending for some time. It was agreed, without her son's prior knowledge, that the headmaster would inform all the boys at the school's assembly the next morning of her son's condition. They both felt this would benefit her son making life easier for him him at school. Before the announcement very few of the other boys had even noticed, and the result was that instantly, much to her son's embarrassment, everyone knew he was a sufferer of psoriasis.

The moral of this story is: make sure your child is informed and you both agree to any decisions you make regarding their welfare, as it's your child who will have to cope with the results.

## Case histories

A child of five and a half was brought to see us by her mother. Her psoriasis had developed very suddenly at the age of one year old. It appeared that the onset of her psoriasis occurred just a few days after her mother had explained to her that in a few months' time she would have a baby brother or sister. It appeared on her body and her face, and the biggest problem for both the parents and the child was the severity of the irritation. Her percentage of coverage was about 25% at the time of her visit.

We talked to the mother and the child together and separately and the mother revealed that the girl was wonderful to her new sister, looked after her, cuddled her and was like a little mother. The child told the therapist that she really loved her little sister.

The irritation of her skin was causing loss of sleep for all the family. The Mora-Therapy test showed that her lungs and digestive system were particularly weak. Also, there was an imbalance in the nervous system. Psychologically we interpreted that as 'something she was unable to express' (lungs) and 'something she could not digest' (digestion). In Greek medicine, the intestines are called the seat of our emotions.

Our recommendation was that she take some gentle fruit, flower and plant remedies, spray Evian water on the skin and apply a homoeopathic cream to help relieve the irritation. It was also recommended that some lavender oil was added to her bath water.

It was explained to the mother that the child was showing signs of fear and insecurity. The mother was advised to show the child as much love and affection as possible as, although she was showing signs of accepting and loving her sister, deep inside her she was carrying suppressed emotions that she was unable to express or even recognise, and they were affecting the condition of her skin.

We arranged for our resident aromatherapist and masseur to teach the mother how to massage her daughter in order to help to re-bond them. Seven weeks later, the child was 100% clear of her psoriasis. This was in June 1989, and to our knowledge she is still clear today.

A 10-year-old boy, with scalp psoraisis and lesions on his lower legs, came to see us with his parents. He had taken a long course of antibiotics when he was one year old for sinus problems.

Eight years later, whilst playing sports at school, he was kicked in the kidneys and severely bruised. Very shortly after his psoriasis appeared. The Mora-Therapy test showed his kidneys were badly out of balance and his lungs showed a weakness. The large intestines and the liver were also affected.

He was recommended to add a drink made from plant extract and a fruit extract remedy every day to aid the detoxification of the kidneys, and a few drops of flower essences were suggested to help him release the shock that he had experienced two years previously. Interestingly enough, his skin needed a special natural cream that is more often recommended for bruising.

Five weeks later, the internal organs of the body showed a dramatic improvement. For example the reading on his lungs were 69 on the initial consultation, after the second visit they showed a reading of 49 but his skin showed very little improvement. He was asked to continue on the same treatment for a further two months when he then showed a 100% clearance of his psoriasis, which was in the spring of 1989.

If your child is a skin sufferer, be heartened: there is safe, natural effective help available that will help them to recover their health. The holistic apporoach to healing the skin, based on the principles of holistic medicine, will prove to be a worthy investment into your child's future.

# Chapter 10

# Coping as a teenager

The years of adolescence are not without stresses and can be one of the most difficult phases for a young person to pass through unscathed. For a teenager with psoriasis the experiences that await you at this time in your life, which lasts for about eight to ten years, are nothing like you knew as a child. Those twilight years between leaving childhood behind and not quite being accepted as an adult seem to take a long time to pass. Your parents and other authority figures expect you to act like an adult with no previous experience or guidance, and all you have as examples are those very people around you whose own behaviour can often leave something to be desired.

Nothing prepares you for being catapulted into your teenage years – ones which should represent maturity, fun, freedom to have your own choices, a little independence and some respect. Instead, many of you will have to deal with all manner of confusing situations and emotions. At home you often have the family pressures as they reluctantly release you from their grip. Your wings will be spreading by the time your parents are in their early forties if they married young. If your mother is eager to return to work she will feel a new found freedom, that you are now able to look after yourself more and don't need to be so dependent on her. Perhaps you will even be earning a little money of your own. This could mean that, with your new-career-minded mother, you suddenly feel abandoned, let down, like she cares more for her own needs than yours.

Do you have to return home from school or work with no-one at home to greet you, or do you stay out until someone is in the house before you get home? Perhaps you enjoy this new-found peace, and prefer to be alone for a few hours each day. Are you expected to help with the household chores much more than previously, do the shopping, run errands or look after younger members of the family? Whatever new responsibilities you have been allocated, unless you want to leave home at an early age, accept them with good grace, and discuss with the family anything you feel is unfair or unreasonable. Why? Because, if you don't, your psoriasis will worsen even more quickly as you cope with other changes that are about to take place.

Your physical body will be developing as well as your mental capacity. Some of these changes may seem bewildering if you don't understand what is happening to you and what to expect. Your pace of life on an every-day basis will quicken as more and more avenues and opportunities become available to you. The pressures of achieving academic qualifications and making career choices will present themselves. You may view your parents with suspicion, distrust and often resentment at what may be their lack of understanding and support during these years. You are convinced you know what is best for you, but they insist that only they do, and all the while you are living under their roof and they are paying your way, they persist in making decisions on your behalf.

Who do you turn to at these difficult times? There really is no-one is there?

Your friends are the same age and can only agree with you as they are normally going through the same process, and your parents and other family members either don't want to understand or have really forgotten their teenage years and how they dealt with them.

Some of you, I am sure, have understanding, supportive parents who will be able to take you every step of the way. Other parents do understand and want to help, but teenagers are afraid to ask for advice or support for fear of rejection or ridicule, or just because they don't want to admit they need help. Are you guilty of that? If so, try changing, and you will really notice a difference in the condition of your skin.

## Skin changes

The skin changes during the teenage years. Some will experience the onset of psoriasis around this time and must learn to manage it as soon as possible. Sweating and greasiness can occur and you must be scrupulous in cleanliness, taking regular showers and changing your clothes, perhaps more than once a day, especially underwear. Acne, boils, eczema, warts, athlete's foot, chilblains, psoriasis, pityriasis, dandruff and ringworm of the groin can all be associated with the onset of puberty. Don't despair, it will pass.

As you are going through such a long complex series of experiences you will need to pay attention to your energy levels. Young people do not necessarily have more energy than older people. It is something you have to work at, and it can be achieved by paying attention to the foods you eat, and learning to deal with stress. The stress of going through this emergence into a new life can leave you feeling exhausted. It can become too much bother to keep your room tidy, pick your clothes up, too lazy to read or study, and your parents' attitude to these problems may not help you. If so, it will only be because they do not understand that this is not rebellion or disrespect for them and the rest of the family, but rather just something that is happening to you because of the factors associated with puberty and adolescence. Help them to understand for all your sakes. Don't assume that, because they are your parents, they should know or remember. It is important to your psoriasis and your health to gain their understanding and support during this trying time.

Study the science of nutrition and your skin, and the value of healthy eating. It will make so much difference to the quality of your future and help you to pass through your teenage years with the minimum of health problems.

Try to be aware of any changes in your behaviour patterns especially if they are likely to create a revolution at home, school or university. There is some glandular activity that takes place in your body that directs your development during this time. Signs of anxiety can appear. Some will be about what is happening to you on a physical and psychological level, others will be concerning the subject of sex, and what is going on in the world. You may be worrying about your future, what career to choose, what subjects to study, and many many more will emerge over these years as new challenges present themselves, new opportunities arise and choices are to be made. Tell yourself you are embarking on an interesting voyage of discovery, and acquire the ability to laugh, especially at yourself, when you experience embarrassing or awkward situations. It really can save you.

Boredom is something you may encounter as you leave behind your childhood pursuits and look for more stimulating adult activities. The need for privacy will become more apparent and it is important to mention this to your family when it occurs in order to avoid confrontations when you prefer to stay on your own away from family or social gatherings.

## Self-consciousness

Self-consciousness will also be something you may suffer from and it could affect you more strongly because of your psoriasis. If you decide to take up sports in an attempt to gain some exercise there is a coverage cream available that comes in different skin shades, especially developed for psoriasis sufferers. It is totally waterproof so will allow you to play tennis or go swimming, or whatever you choose. This will help deal with some of the self-consciousness.

If you are worrying if you will ever be able to clear your skin, the answer is that it is both possible to relieve your condition dramatically, and learn to control it and prevent it from worsening.

It is also possible to clear it. We do not use the word 'cure' because that means permanent, 'clear' is more realistic. You can read the case histories in this book. The most effective way to deal with your skin is to try to forget you suffer, and concentrate your mind on other things, helping others or planning your future.

To put your mind at rest and to illustrate that there really is genuine help available I am going to tell you about a case of a young teenager who consulted the Centre for help. There follows the letter she wrote us:

Dear Sandra

I am sorry it has taken me so long to finally sit down and write this letter but I have been rather busy lately with my mock exams [which she passed]. My psoriasis appeared when I was eight years old, shortly after the death of my grandmother. I went from the doctor to the specialist, trying every kind of cream under the sun without success. Although my psoriasis was distressing them it wasn't until I became older that it really upset me.

When I was fourteen I went on an exchange visit with my school to Germany. I remember dragging my mum around every single clothes shop in the town trying to find a 'suitable' swimming costume, i.e. one with a high neck so that it would cover up my chest and back. It was a long search – you don't find many costumes like that.

When I was fifteen I took part in a gang show, I was in the dance line and one evening whilst trying on costumes, one of the dancers screamed with horror: 'God, what's that all over your arms?' Of course, by now I had learnt my answer by heart and everyone was amazed at how 'it didn't bother me'. However, that night at home I broke down in front of my mum, which is something I rarely did because it upset my parents, since they felt so helpless, and even responsible. My mum put her arms around me, and I asked her how she could bear to look or touch my skin. After all I couldn't bear to look at or touch my skin, so how could someone else?

I then tried various other treatments such as using a PUVA sunbed and trying a vitamin diet which resulted in me replacing two meals a day with a powdered drink, and taking 24 capsule-sized tablets a day – consequently I began to go home for dinner instead of eating in the school canteen. When all this failed I resigned myself to the fact that I was stuck with my psoriasis, long sleeves, trousers and high collars were here to stay, and boyfriends were definitely out.

Today, two years after I went to The Alternative Centre, my skin is clear. I admit I still have the odd red spot or two, but nowadays, at 18, real spots are more of a problem. More importantly, during the past two years I have learnt that my psoriasis didn't bother other people, just myself.

I have decided that you can add my name to this letter, if you feel it appropriate, simply because I feel that if I didn't want my name to be written, it would look as though I was ashamed of my psoriasis and what I have been through, as I think that would be a bad example for other sufferers.

I would just like to finish by saying thank you to you, and everyone else at The Alternative Centre who have helped me, for your patience and understanding.

I hope you are all fit and well.

Donna Hunt (18)

I know Donna will not mind me telling you that she succeeded in passing her exams without the usual flare up with her psoriasis and is now studying hard to go to University to study modern languages.

Donna went through the holistic programme for psoriasis and was taught relaxation techniques to practise after her studying each night to restore her peace of mind before sleeping. It helped to relieve some of the anxiety associated with exams and was a valuable contributory factor to her skin remaining clear during this stressful time.

Another young lady, who has asked to be named is Karla Jeffs and her letter reads:

Dear Toni

I can't wait to tell you how pleased I was to be asked to write to you and let you know all the benefits I had for my skin after visiting. When I first came to you my skin was so bad that the only place I did not have psoriasis was on the palms of my hands and the soles of my feet. Jane gave me all the natural remedies I needed and told me to start using the Pharbifarm formulas 1 and 2, with the shampoo. This was a great help and I found it very soothing.

Within a week I was noticing a difference, the pain was easier and the flaking was not so bad. Anne had also told me about my diet and advised me on all the foods I could avoid.

After a month I saw Sylvia, who started healing me. It was with this as well as all the other treatments that my skin really started to improve. I was now beginning to wear short sleeved tops and feel much more confident about myself. It's almost a year now since I came to you and I really know that without all your help I would still be suffering. I just hope I can keep my skin under control by myself without worrying about it as I did before.

I really am very grateful to you for everything you have done for me, many thanks once again.

Believe me these are not just rare examples of success. We have seen many cases like this over the past ten years. So you see, there is no reason why your psoriasis should add to your problems of being a teenager.

Teenagers, though, do spend a great deal of time brooding over their physical and health problems, but seldom know how to do anything about them. Unless you have the financial resources to pay for treatments, consultations, books and creams, you are very much at the mercy of your parents, and if they are not as supportive as the parents of these two young people whose letters you have just read, you often have no choice but to remain with the orthodox treatments until you can take care of your own needs. If this is the case, telephone the Alternative Centre after you have read this book. You may find you can gain all the information you need to help yourself. If not, write to me personally.

You really can help your skin to heal without spending a great deal of money. This book will help you.

## *Psychological problems*

Some of the psychological problems you will experience whilst being a teenager will need some understanding. The first step is to recognize the symptoms and accept they are a natural part of growing up, so that there is no need to reproach yourself or feel unusual, guilty or frightened.

There is a certain fear attached to the process of growing up. Stepping out into the unknown, into an alien world of hidden experiences, yet to be discovered, some being wonderful, some disturbing, some confusing, some enlightening. This journey will seem somewhat like being in the centre of a maze, offering a series of alternative routes that will try to fool you into taking different directions, each one seeming to be the right one, giving you the impression that you have different routes to choose from. But don't be fooled, these distractions are there to test you.

There is only one route for you can take – the right one. Which one will that be? Trust your intuition, and you will find the right road. In other words there will be lots of temptations for you to fall into and some of the psychological factors you will experience can influence your decisions. So, be aware. You are being tested, and you can pass with flying colours. What will these temptations be? Well, they could be drugs, smoking, drinking, sexual promiscuity, none of which will benefit your long-term health, even if you only experiment temporarily.

There is also a choice of characteristics you can develop that will also have no benefit to your future, such as greed, selfishness and bitterness. My point is that you can learn to control your habits and personality traits at your age, just the same as you can learn to take care of your health. This way you will ensure that you will be able to pave your way to a happy, healthy life. So, pay attention to the risks that await you in your youth. Learn to recognize some of the processes you are going through, and to interpret what they mean in psychological terms. For example, any form of idol or hero worship as with pop stars, cult figures, film stars is associated with a fear of emotional security. If you prefer to stay at home instead of mixing with friends, you could have an underlying fear of growing up. If you are suffering from these symptoms, try a hostelling trek, or volunteer for social work and spend some time helping those less fortunate.

If you sense you are very sensitive and touchy, perhaps more than you feel you should be, this could be a symptom of lack of confidence and attention. Try offering to help more at home or at school events. This normally helps.

Feeling fed up with life, can happen even when you have not been alive for very long. Coupled with morbid anxiety this can cause depression. What you must do is accept that it is a temporary phase and often comes when you cannot foresee the future. Introduce a little light-heartedness and humour into your life. It can work wonders.

Phobias are a symptom of setting your standards too high, or perhaps your parents are making excessive demands of you. I have heard so many cases of this with counselling, so you are not alone.

Anorexia nervosa is a chronic serious slimming disease that can be life-threatening. It occurs more in girls than boys, although they can become victims also. Drastic weight loss is experienced as a result of severe appetite loss. It makes you very depressed, very unattractive in appearance and behaviour, and very ill. Psychologically, it is associated with wanting the world to be a perfect clean place, an inability to accept life or yourself. Physically it can be treated successfully with zinc therapy and counselling, and homoeopathic treatment. So don't ignore, or try to hide, this problem if you feel it occurring.

## Sex

One word of advice, don't be too eager to experiment because you will be very disappointed, despite remarks from your friends. Why? Because sex goes together with love, and it is not really recommended as being worthwhile without it. Also, denying yourself until you are in a loving relationship does not mean you are going to miss out. Sex will always be there. But it should be something we deserve, an expression of love, not something we have a right to. The act of love must be treated with care and respect. It is not something you experiment with, like learning to swim, because it involves another human being, someone else's emotions.

Be patient, the opportunity will be there, when you are ready and find the right person for a long-term relationship. You are different, responsible and caring, you are also a psoriasis sufferer, which makes you a very special person in terms of sensitivity, and many other special qualities we know are exclusive to skin sufferers.

Your psoriasis will certainly not respond well if you have any guilty secrets, any worries or secret liaisons. Your parents trust you to be responsible and have a sense of right and wrong. So, don't let them down, you will only let yourself down, and your psoriasis will react. Be patient, sensible, and prepare for your future, everything will follow.

Being a teenager can be fun, your last personal little piece of freedom before you enter the real world, the world of professional and financial responsibilities, marriage, children. So make the most of the time and, above all, take care of your psoriasis.

---

# Chapter 11

# The effects on family life

When any member of the family suffers from any form of handicap, it inevitably affects family life. Resentment and jealousy can occur with partners, and other members of the family as a result of the attention the sufferer demands, through no fault of their own. This is a particular problem for parents with children with psoriasis. The sufferer, in turn, senses the resentment which increases the severity of the skin problem.

Recognizing these symptoms in a child's behaviour can be difficult, and correcting these behavioural patterns may mean enlisting professional help. The reactions are not always directed towards the source of resentment. These could be playing truant from school, temper tantrums, not eating, feigning illness, constant rudeness, stealing, lying and many other unacceptable tendencies. This pattern of behaving often carried out by the brothers or sisters of the suffering child, is a deliberate aim of diverting your attention away from the child who needs it. It is important for the welfare of everyone in a family that the child or children in question is confronted as to the real reasons for any unruly or inconsiderate behaviour.

Be sure to give them the confidence and security and love that will enable them to reveal the true reasons for their behaviour. Ask questions. Do they resent the time, money or attention spent on the sufferer? Don't chastise them for saying how they feel. We are all guilty of withholding our true feelings, and this can cause unnecessary stress. Normally this habit, that stays with us for life, comes from holding back as a child, which blocks us from fully expressing our emotions. Then we are unable to heal our pain by sharing it, and in fear we keep it to ourselves.

Unless your children are secure and feel safe to express their real feelings the behaviour patterns will continue and the child that is a sufferer will feel even more isolated and guilty that they could be the cause. Needless to say if this happens the family are in danger of having to deal with even more complex problems than just a child with psoriasis.

There follows a very tragic story of what happened to one family because of their inability to recognize and solve a problem of resentment in their other children. This is not a case of psoriasis but anorexia nervosa, and it is an example of what illness can do to a family if not handled correctly by the parents or with the help of professionals.

The parents, who were relatively young in their early forties, had three daughters of 26, 14 and 16. The eldest one became a victim of anorexia nervosa, the slimming disease, in her late teens, much to the shock of her parents. They struggled to help her recover and she was hospitalized on more than one occasion when her weight became dangerously low. During the years she was a sufferer she got married to a very nice young man determined to help her.

Whilst the parents were paying so much attention to their eldest daughter which involved the mother staying in London, away from the family home, often they did not notice the resentment building up in the other two daughters, in particular the 16-year-old. Both of the daughters were beginning to show signs of disturbed, rebellious behaviour, but the parents were so obviously preoccupied with the eldest daughter who was becoming more ill every day. It was only for a wonderful specialist who was helping her maintain her will to live that she lived as long as she did. Yes, she died at the age of 26, much to the distress of her parents and husband.

During the last months of her illness, neither of the other daughters showed obvious signs of concern for the suffering of their sister, and their behaviour was worsening and taking the form of aggression and rudeness to the very unhappy and distressed parents who, because of their grief and tragedy, were having their own set of personal problems within their relationship.

The mother told me it was as though her daughters were punishing them for loving and caring for the eldest daughter and resented the care they had to take of her, one daughter said: 'I'll be glad when she dies.' Within months after her elder daughter was buried I was told by a close friend of hers that the 16-year-old was now developing symptoms of anorexia nervosa and making herself ill; perhaps in an attempt to get attention. The next news I received, a year or so later, was the youngest daughter was also developing signs of becoming anorexic.

I met the parents just after their latest news and the mother was close to breakdown, and was still grieving for the eldest daughter. The husband, a patient, gentle soul, was at a loss to know what to do to save what was left of his family. The wife was also coping with unpleasant symptoms of menopause, and their marriage, what was left of it, was now in name only.

This is an extreme case I know but just shows you how resentment, anger and bitterness can arise when one child is sick and what the results can be.

The just and most practical step you can take is to explain to other children everything they should know about psoriasis. Teach them all the precautions and treatments, and food guidelines and let the child who is suffering explain how he or she feels, without you interrupting in order to protect.

Allow the others to participate so that everyone can become more tolerant and gain a better understanding of how everyone feels. Teaching children about the importance of other people's feelings and needs at an early age is far more important than we appreciate. Sometimes the sheer pace of our lives distracts us from what really is essential and we overlook or do not make time for teaching children, and preparing them for some of the emotional and psychological obstacles they will have to overcome.

When you are having to deal with delicate, sensitive situations, cast your mind back to when you were a child. Children possess the same emotions that we do but they are more intense, much more vulnerable and more sensitive, especially if they suffer from psoriasis. Can you remember your feelings of shyness, rejection, embarrassment, fear, shame and loneliness? Well, most children experience those feelings every day, but don't communicate them to us, often because they don't know how.

By becoming aware that your psoriasis suffering member of the family is dealing with their own set of problems, and treating them with care you will help eliminate resentment from others, and the rewards will be beneficial to the welfare and happiness of all of you.

Children have to be taught how to bring out the best in others, as do adults. We all have good points and those points are not always obvious. Education in human relations is far more important than all the subjects learnt at school, and the place to start teaching them is in the home as soon as they are old enough.

Every effort must be made to create and maintain peace and harmony in the house. Not an easy task, by any means, but a worthwhile one, and one that usually rests with the mother of the household. This is not to say that the father should be exempt from contributing, but generally we have to accept that women are better at public relations.

It takes a great deal of understanding and support to successfully raise a child with a handicap and the most common complaints I receive from women is that they wish their husbands would be more supportive. To be fair to the male members of the household, they may well be the sole breadwinner and having to continually finance everyone's needs, including the latest discoveries in 'miracle cures' for the sufferer. Just because your husband doesn't express how he feels does not mean he is uncaring, indifferent or insensitive to what is going on around him. It just means he is unable to contribute in many other ways than by providing the money to feed, clothe, school and provide for his family. Not an easy task to keep up with as most men will agree.

It is surprising what a lonely place marriage can be, especially if your child gains more attention than your partner because of their skin condition. We live behind our permanent masks of control, not showing or saying what we feel, holding back pain, as we learnt as children. If we feel resentment towards our handicapped child this is felt as unnatural, and very selfish. But it is normal, and there should be no self reproach. If one partner feels resentment towards the other because their needs are not being met, this can lead to them looking elsewhere for the comfort they need. The likely consequences of this are broken marriages, and children with psoriasis suffer badly from separation or divorce problems, particularly as they escalate the condition.

The boy was eight years old when he came to see me with his parents. They said his condition had become very severe when the father had moved out. It had spread to his face, which caused him considerable distress as he was the only child at school who suffered. The parents decided to reconcile for the sake of the boy, and have succeeded in re-capturing some of the love, intimacy and friendship they felt they had lost. It can take a lot of effort to save your marriage, but it is worthwhile. Sharing a history with someone you decided to marry because you loved them. Having a change of heart about how to treat them, making time for a little romance and time together, and not being afraid to let them see the real you in terms of feelings, all adds up to saving your marriage. Coping with children with psoriasis, being a one parent family, the traumas of divorce and all the emotional and practical upheavals associated with splitting the family is enough reason to try to resolve your differences.

The happier you are, the better you feel about yourself, and the happier all those around you will feel. Frequently I have to persuade patients, women in particular, to enjoy being selfish without feeling guilt. There is always a conflict. Mothers or wives who are psoriasis sufferers are even reluctant to prepare their food separately from the family. They seem unable to contemplate even allowing half an hour per day to relax in order to help heal their skin.

How can it be selfish to want to be well enough to enjoy your partner and family? Parents who are psoriasis sufferers know the condition can sometimes make them feel edgy, irritable and bad tempered. Isn't that being more selfish than just taking a little more time and care for yourself to improve your condition?

Some patients have told me they have deliberately chosen careers that meant they could live away from their families because their psoriasis creates such a problem for them. Don't let your condition, or the psoriasis of your child, run your life. It really is unnecessary. The best way to avoid this is to learn as much as you can about self-help therapies. You will then feel more in control, which will improve relations within family life, and certainly with your partner. You are really being more selfish using your psoriasis as an excuse to avoid issues, than taking some time to get well.

Men are usually the most reluctant to begin treatment, but when they decide to take action they really are a pleasure to deal with. In my experience, once a man makes up his mind to take charge of his health, he will seldom deviate from the programme. Their approach is very straightforward and businesslike, and providing you explain in logical terms, although they take longer than women initially, they persist with treatment until they achieve the success they expect. Women, on the other hand, are quicker to respond to the suggestion of trying to clear their skin or improve their health, but often experience a series of false starts whilst their emotions argue with their logic.

There seems to be more fear of becoming well with women than men, perhaps because they fear their lives will change. They may be pressured to return to work or be expected to respond in other ways. This becomes most obvious when the skin is beginning to show signs of healing. You can sense the inner conflict in some patients as they are battling within with the question of whether they really want to clear their psoriasis! What will it mean? Will it mean all those around them will expect more?

Men seem to respond more easily to suggestions for helping to improve a marriage, and on how to introduce romance – maybe because of the financial cost of divorce. When advice is given to some of our lady patients on how to be more romantic and revive their marriage, you can sense a feeling that this is something the men should be doing with chocolates, flowers, expensive gifts and candlelight dinners.

There are many ways to improve your marriage romantically, and plenty of books to help you, and I feel it is necessary for us all to learn as much as we can about how to make the people we love feel special. It is often something we forget to do, especially if we are married, in a long-term relationship, or are preoccupied with our own psoriasis or that of our children.

It is difficult to share the life of a psoriasis sufferer, even more so if they have given up themselves. Living with someone with an incurable illness can feel like a life sentence. There are times when you just want to run away, but feel too guilty or sorry for your partner. I think one of the hardest things to cope with is the mood swings which result from how their skin feels.

Sleeping with a sufferer is not always pleasant and of course sexual relations can be a problem because of how the sufferer feels about themselves, or purely because they feel so uncomfortable and their skin is so painful.

If your partner suffers it is important to ask them to explain how they feel. If they cannot tell you, ask them to write it down, it is wonderful therapy and will help both of you. Be patient with the moods, and be mature enough to understand they are not directed at you, it's because sufferers feel so bad about themselves, get angry, and frustrated because they feel so trapped in their skin.

There are actually many ways you can help them achieve a better quality of life. The one thing everyone needs most of all is moral support and love. Don't bully, shout, be angry or try to make decisions on their behalf without the sufferer's knowledge. You cannot force a sufferer to get well just because it will help *you*. Some don't want to get well. That is their right. Then you just have to make the decision about whether you want to stay in the relationship. Don't emotionally blackmail or pressure with ultimatums. However you feel, your partner feels worse.

One partner I counselled whilst abroad told me how her psoriasis-suffering husband, who also suffered from arthritis, drove her to distraction with his psoriasis because he would not give up the foods she knew were bad for him, in particular chocolate which made him itch, especially at night. She had a very loud voice, and we were in a hotel lounge with her husband sitting close by listening to her complaints. This is not the normal place to see patients, but I had no choice because she insisted I talk to her there and then. As the evening went on she became more and more agitated because her husband would not come over and see me to talk about how he could clear his skin. He was quite happily playing cards with friends. I felt instinctively that his psoriasis bothered the wife more than the sufferer, which is often the case.

I confronted her with this, and she agreed, adding she hated all the dead skin in the bed every morning. I then asked her if her husband had been a psoriasis sufferer when they married. Apparently he had. I then told her that her husband could not cure his psoriasis just to make her feel better, so she had two options – either she left him, or stayed with him and learned how to live with psoriasis, as she was probably causing her partner more stress with her unrealistic demands than the psoriasis itself. Three years later I met the sufferer, and he told me his wife had left him, and that his psoriasis had improved dramatically!

Another case of how others can affect the sufferer is of a young man from New York who came to see us a few years ago in a state of great distress. He told us that he was 95 per cent covered in psoriasis and had been travelling around the world to find a cure. He was due to be married in just three months and the family of the bride had told him he must be clear of psoriasis for the wedding night. It did not matter if the psoriasis returned after that night. The bride did not mind whether he had psoriasis when they got married. Can you imagine the anxiety level and despair of this sad man? It was further aggravated because it was an arranged marriage. We could only explain to him that we could try, but because his stress was so high and he was only visiting London for one day we could not make any promises. This was many years before we perfected the holistic approach which might have made it possible.

If you have never shared your life with a sufferer, be prepared, it can change your life considerably. Taking a trip to the Dead Sea in Israel, where you can both enjoy a good holiday and clear their skin is a marvellous investment for both of you. Then you can learn how to prevent your partner's psoriasis returning. The UVB home-use unit will make a difference to both of your lives also. Be sure never to be seen as more concerned or less concerned about your partner's condition than they are. An accurate assessment of your partner's character and personality will help you to handle them in the best way for both of you.

It is a common mistake to make the assumption that when we meet someone suffering from a handicap, they will automatically respond to your help and encouragement to heal their skin. But the truth about psoriasis sufferers is that they have often lived with their condition so long they cannot visualize life without it, especially if every previous effort has failed, or they have an underlying psychological reason for holding on to it. Some just cannot face the thought of further wasted efforts, or spending any more money on 'miracle cures'.

One of the most difficult things for a non-sufferer to grasp is how someone cannot possibly want to get rid of something that looks so unpleasant and is so painful and uncomfortable. The truth of the matter is that most do, but in their own time. They always do try another treatment at some time, but they can only cope with paying so much attention to their skin.

Each time they treat it, it brings to the surface a complex of emotions about how they feel about themselves. It reminds them of the suffering, the restrictions, and often they try to forget they have it for a while until it demands they try again. So don't despair, just handle your partner gently. They are not necessarily rejecting your offers of help, they are just rejecting the idea of treating their skin for a while.

The following story illustrates people's different approaches to their problems and may help you to decide what type of person your partner is.

Once upon a time there were two frogs. One was an optimist, of a cheery happy nature, able to see the funny side of everything. The other was a pessimist, gloomy and over-serious. One day they both fell in a milk churn. 'How awful, we'll never get out of here and we cannot survive in milk,' signed the pessimist. 'We are going to die in agony. I don't want to suffer. I would rather kill myself.' He banged his head against the side of the milk churn and sank like a stone. 'Well, I'm not going to commit suicide,' said the optimistic frog. 'If I've got to die I am going to die happy. I shall have at least one last fling.' With these words the optimist began splashing around, dancing, singing and laughing. After a while he noticed that his exuberant movements were turning the milk into butter. Soon he was able to climb out and leap to safety.

How your partner chooses to manage their psoriasis will affect your life, and progressively more so if they have a negative approach to their problem. The daily ritual of applying treatments, precautions that have to be taken with food, careful planning for holidays and your social arrangements cannot fail to affect you.

We have spoken to families who have never had a holiday, the children never knowing what building sand castles feels like, because of the reluctance of the sufferer to expose themselves to the sun on a beach. One patient from South America told me how his psoriasis didn't seem to affect his children too much until they wanted him to teach them to swim.

In most cases it is not the psoriasis of the partner that is a problem but how they handle it. Beware of the demands for attention that you may not be giving so often. Because you are used to your partner's condition, sometimes they want you to suffer because they are suffering. Other times they are saying: 'Please understand how I am suffering'.

General morale can become very low and it will affect you.

If you want to make the relationship work, be sure your partner does too and will contribute towards life. Don't forget to pay compliments, show affection, keep your sense of humour and help them see the funnier side of life. Be prepared to enjoy some activities alone, rather than build up resentment within yourself. Resentfulness will not do your health any good or your partner's. But, be careful to handle this independence carefully. Perhaps your partner will decide to join you when their skin is healed. Your patience, moral support, common sense and humour will help both your partner and your family enjoy the quality of life you all deserve, despite psoriasis.

---

# Chapter 12

# PMT, pregnancy and menopause

A great deal of distress can be caused by an imbalance of a woman's hormones associated with premenstrual tension, pregnancy and the menopause. This can affect behaviour, causing tearfulness, argumentativeness, feelings of insecurity, and sometimes violence. Many women are unaware that they have a hormonal imbalance, or how it affects their health. It can occur without warning, and not only creates havoc in the lives of sufferers, but also for those around them.

Psoriasis sufferers nearly always experience a worsening of the skin during this time, and it happens from teenagers, who have just started their monthly menstrual cycle, to older women beginning menopause. Many sufferers explain that they feel so depressed and helpless at this time, not only because they have hormonal changes but because their skin appears to become more angry and painful.

## *PMT*

In the case of premenstrual tension there is a great deal you can do to minimise the effect of premenstrual tension on the mind and the body which automatically will help your psoriasis. With nutritional enhancements, either by way of introducing certain foods into your daily diet before your period is due, or by taking supplements, some of these discomforting symptoms can be alleviated. It is, I feel, preferable to obtain the vitamins and minerals you need from the food you eat rather than take them as individual supplements. This, of course, is not always possible, and in such cases supplements are invaluable.

A zinc deficiency is a common factor in premenstrual tension, and your iron levels can be depleted if you are a heavy tea or coffee drinker. Liver, in meat or tablet form, kidneys, dried peaches, prunes, molasses, dried beans, raisins, egg-yolks and green leafy vegetables are high in iron. It is advisable for vitamin E and C to be taken with the foods to help absorption. Zinc is contained in meat, fish, brewer's yeast, dried legumes, pumpkin seeds, egg-yolks and milk.

Magnesium is another trace element that can become deficient during your monthly period. This is available from a natural supplement called dolomite, and also from nuts, apples, raw wheatgerm, green vegetables, figs, yellow corn, lemons and grapefruit.

One of the best ways to avoid premenstrual problems is to increase your calcium intake, as we lose calcium during this time in the month, and this can cause problems sleeping and affect the nerves. Either take a water-soluble calcium supplement for ten days leading up to your period, or eat peeled almonds, soaked in almond oil or plain, every day. Drinking celery juice for 7 days before also helps to relieve the water retention so many women experience. This can either be as soup or as a cold drink to which you can add carrots or watercress.

One of the 'life savers' is the Efamol Evening Primrose Pre-menstrual Pack, available from most health stores and pharmacies. If you suffer from cramps and tiredness, ginger tea can be effective. It helps the back, glands and the nerves. For weakness or dizziness, a wonderful energy booster is to take two tablespoons of raw sesame oil each day for a few days before your period starts. Cutting down on salt will help a great deal in preventing bloating, swelling of the abdomen and breasts.

The monthly periods of a woman are an expression of femininity and fertility, and we are at the absolute mercy of this rhythm. We wonder what symptoms each month will bring, how they will affect our moods and our skin. How will we cope with the pain? What shall we try this time? What a burden we have to bear. We have to totally surrender to this act of nature that is placed upon us, and deal with it as best we can.

Self-surrender is a truly feminine quality. A woman truly happy in her feminine role (and an amazing amount are not) will never feel that she is inferior in any way. It is a failure to feel comfortable and happy as a female that is the root cause of most menstrual problems. Having to go along with what is happening to our bodies and the self-surrender process that the monthly period demands, means letting go. We are, in fact, surrendering part of ourselves as the menstruation is both a 'little birth' and a 'little pregnancy'. For those with menstrual problems there is often an unconscious process within that is refusing to let go, not wanting to surrender, not only to menstruation, but perhaps to sex as well.

By understanding your condition, and taking the necessary precautions to avoid the negative effects of premenstrual tension, you can prevent your psoriasis causing an added unwelcome problem each month.

## *Pregnancy*

Pregnancy can also affect your psoriasis, but not always in a negative way. I have heard of sufferers becoming clear on falling pregnant, and remaining clear throughout the time they are carrying the child. Mostly, though, the psoriasis returns after a couple of months; and sometimes it can be worse than before. Other sufferers tell of their condition remaining the same, getting no worse or no better, and some report a worsening of the condition. This could be due to an increased excretion of progesterone which occurs during pregnancy. Of course there are also many physical and emotional changes that take place in a woman during pregnancy which can influence the skin.

One of the most important requirements is to gain as much knowledge as possible about what is happening to you. This involves all the physical changes, both positive and negative, and the psychological process. This will help you to eliminate any problems that are associated with the pregnancy itself, and your psoriasis. A healthy diet, preferably started before you became pregnant, is one of the most important self-help measures. Basically, the same diet as recommended in the Food Factors chapter is a good guideline.

The most important time for starting a healthy eating regime and relaxation therapy is three months before you conceive, both for you and your partner. This will definitely help in preventing some of the common problems associated with pregnancy.

## *Menopause*

The menopause may not have to be the traumatic and distressing mid-life crisis that we hear of.

This time of our lives is associated with losing our femininity, the diminishing of our sexuality, the mood swings we can expect, the depression, and coping with the empty nest syndrome. The talk is of wrinkling skin, sagging breasts, increased weight, loss of libido. We may also expect to experience hair loss, decalcification of the bones, or even losing partners to younger women. What a depressing picture!

However, it is not all bad news and concentrating on the benefits will help to overcome some of the physical symptoms that we have little control over. First, we no longer have to endure monthly periods, and we can enjoy sex without fear of pregnancy; the experience of children leaving home can become a wonderful experience of freedom. No longer are you tied to the home and demands of family life. Instead, there are a wealth of opportunities to study, to work, to develop skills that you may have abandoned years ago.

All these factors will affect your skin, but by following the holistic approach to psoriasis you will be able to minimize your suffering. You will be able to enjoy the spontaneity of life, perhaps for the first time in many years. Many post-menopausal women discover that they are more creative. Think of it as a re-birthing process. You will now give birth to new ideas and new concepts.

# Success stories and letters

Miss X was seven years old when her psoriasis began. Her legs, arms, body and face were affected. Excess scratching had caused the skin to bleed on many occasions. Her chest, which was covered in psoriasis caused this young girl, now 15, great distress.

In this case it was difficult to pinpoint what triggered her psoriasis. All her elimination organs showed with the Mora-therapy test that they were overburdened. So, she was asked to embark on a detoxification programme designed specially for her needs.

Her psoriasis improved so much on the programme that she did not return until ten months later for a check up. During this time she continued her treatment at home, and just re-ordered supplies when she needed them.

On her initial consultation the Mora reading for her skin had been 39. On her second visit it had registered 53, which was an excellent improvement. As her skin began to clear she became a victim of bulimia, an unpleasant eating disorder involving bingeing and subsequent self-inflicted vomiting. She had successfully hidden this complaint from her parents but had decided to confess to us on her second consultation, and asked for help.

It was recommended that she take some natural food supplements to help repair the organs of her body affected by this disorder. Spiritual healing and counselling was also suggested, and through this it was discovered that her psoriasis had started when her grandmother had died.

The natural grieving process had been blocked in her parents' attempt to protect her, as she was only seven years old at the time her grandmother died. The sessions of healing and counselling, along with her holistic healing programme for her skin, resulted in the disappearance of her eating disorder and her psoriasis.

Another case was of a lady who has since recovered her health and is now working with handicapped children. Her case involves the effects of amalgam dental fillings, the metals used for filling teeth that can seep into the bloodstream and become absorbed by the body and affect the skin. She was married with two children and had psoriasis on the front of her legs that appeared very raised and stubborn. She had previously been treated by dermatologists and natural medicine with no success. However, after her de-toxification programme her skin appeared to improve a little in that the irritation and sores cleared.

On her second visit to the Centre, it was detected that she had a hormone problem which was having an adverse effect on the condtion of her skin, and it was recommended that she consult a homoeopathic doctor for help in regulating this problem.

Despite some improvement there was still a build-up of toxins in her body, and further investigation revealed that it was due to the highly toxic effect of the fillings in her teeth. She was sent to a specialist for confirmation of this diagnosis, and she was advised to undergo extensive dental treatment involving the replacement of the amalgam fillings with recommended white fillings, whilst continuing with her de-toxification programme.

Over a five month period each filling was replaced. Meanwhile, a close monitoring of the patient's health was carried out at the Centre, with continual modification of the de-toxification programme to keep pace with her healing process. When the last of the dental work had been carried out her skin started to heal.

Another success story is of a young lady who is a professional model who, whilst on a modelling assignment in Hong Kong, contracted severe food poisoning. She was in her early twenties and had been a sufferer from psoriasis since she was nine years old, but it had regularly gone into remission which had allowed her to pursue her chosen career.

The food poisoning caused her skin to react, and she was obviously very distressed as her profession depended very much on her appearance.

The Mora-therapy reading showed a very weak digestive system, so she was recommended to take some natural remedies and homoeopathic treatment to clear the remains of the food poisoning. This patient is now well clear of her psoriasis, and she returned to Hong Kong for another successful assignment, with strict instructions to pay attention to her eating habits, and a list of what foods to avoid.

A young man from New Zealand, who had moved to England, found his skin had become progressively worse since he had been living in London. He was missing the clean air and sunshine, and the slower pace of life in New Zealand, and was having difficulty in adjusting to his new way of life.

After 25 years of living in a relatively unpolluted part of the world, the environmental pollution his skin was now exposed to in England made it even more difficult for him to respond as successfully as he should do to a UVB home-use therapy unit he was using. Tap water was another factor that was detected as slowing his healing process.

It was necessary for a considerable change to be made to his diet, and many suggestions were made on how to avoid the pollution problems. It became clear as treatment progressed that there was heavy metal poisoning in his system, but as it was not possible to detect exactly what the cause was, he was sent for scientific testing. This was after he remembered that he had spent some months working in a mine in Tasmania a few years ago. It was felt that the metal he had been exposed to during this time could be responsible for blocking his self-healing process, as there appeared to have been no other exposure to toxic metals. The tests confirmed that this was the case, as the series of metals he had been exposed to were the ones that came to light. These were silver, tin, copper, zinc, palladium and pewter. Flower essences were recommended, along with a homoeopathic treatment, which were for restoring the muscle tissues, tendons, ligaments and a lack of oxygen which had also been identified. After a few months of treatment this young man was well on the way to clearing his skin, as his body slowly de-toxified.

# *Letters from patients*

**Mrs Moore's story**

My eldest sister (my best friend) died in Cardiff on Good Friday 1984. I spent a lot of time with her and watched with a heavy heart, her descent into dementia. She had always been so elegant, so full of life, so intelligent. She knew me to the end – my voice when she could no longer see, my touch when she could no longer hear. At the other end of the M4 was my husband, retired early after a heart attack and beset with angina and circulation problems. I spent my time between them.

Shortly after my sister died I fell and suffered a severe impacted fracture of the wrist (right arm). Later, on holiday, my psoriasis manifested itself as a very scaley, itchy scalp, and a patch on my right leg, just above the knee, followed by more patches. I was then 66. My doctor shook his head sorrowfully and said 'psoriasis', prescribing the St John Hospital for Skin Diseases Formula for my body and a special shampoo for my scalp.

Things went from bad to worse, and I remember being in a bookshop, opening a book on psoriasis and being so frightened by the very graphic illustrations that I closed it quickly, put it back and ran out of the shop.

At this time my husband was very poorly indeed and we decided to move to Hertfordshire, near my son. I managed to get through the trauma of negotiations and moving, arriving at our new home with a large spare jar of 'dirty looking brown gunge' plus a tube of clean looking cream recommended to me by a fellow sufferer (prescribed by a specialist but obtainable over the counter at our local chemist). I took this cream on holiday that summer and it caused havoc, raising hard carapaces on my upper arms, etc., etc. I was at this time still hobbling badly owing to the severe joint pains, caused by the psoriasis, my doctor had said. I refused all drugs, preferring to hold them in reserve until I really was *in extremis.*

But salvation was at hand! One day, waiting to pay at the local health shop, I picked up a free paper and inside saw an article by Jane Waters on their latest sun canopy. I didn't think we had room for one, but I rang and was told: '. . . there are other things . . . can you come up and talk?' I certainly could, and did. I came back home that afternoon with a light sleep,

Formula 1 and 2, Bath Oil, Shampoo and some good sound advice on diet (which I didn't want to take!). At last, though, there was understanding, warmth and hope.

I improved greatly in general health, but there was something blocking the healing of my skin, and the big breakthrough for me came when Jane's patient probing detected traces of cobalt in my body (a residue of my cobalt cancer treatment in 1964). I was given granules to 'seek and chase out' the errant cobalt, and I began to feel better.

At this time my scalp, ears, back of neck, trunk, arms, legs and toes were a mess. My husband and my two granddaughters (now 7 and 10) had been very supportive although my son and daughter-in-law could not bear to look at the devastated areas. The children inspected my arms every time they saw me, patting my hands gently after pulling down the sleeves of my cotton top again. Their father howled and covered his eyes when I threatened him with a sight of the patches. We had a lot of fun, but seriously, my son said he was very impressed with my general progress.

Jane then passed me on to Dr Bortot, and I am undergoing a gentle cleansing and revitalizing of my whole system. I feel incredibly fit, no joint pains, great easing of the skin, which is now slowly but surely beginning to heal. I sleep well – at one time I used a mini-cradle to keep the clothes off my legs, and to create a large pocket of air around me. I eat well and enjoy every mouthful of my delicious wholemeal bread, my delicious muesli (de luxe, of course!) and the taste of raw cane sugar in my filtered coffee.

I am so grateful to everyone at The Alternative Centre for their care and their friendship, and I am so very grateful for the Prayer for Healing with Laying on of Hands every month at our local church, which has given me the heart to cope with all of this.

## Mrs T writes

It seems as if I have always had psoriasis. In fact I have had it to varying degrees for over twenty years. It started in my early teens on my scalp and then moved to my elbows, knees and back.

I soon found out that the only thing that cleared my condition was the sun. I used to long for the summer when I could sunbathe after school and at weekends. If I was lucky with the weather I could get my skin clear enough by the summer holidays to be able to wear a swimming costume without feeling embarrassed.

In recent years my psoriasis has spread to other parts of my body, and since I started working I have been unable to fit in the necessary sunbathing in my spare time. Instead I have pestered my husband with demands to go somewhere hot and sunny for our holiday. It must be in June so that I can get my skin clear for the rest of the summer, and it must be where we will not meet anyone else we know so that I can be free to sunbathe. While on holiday I am unable to truly relax because I am obsessed with the desire to get enough sun to my body.

I dread having any warm weather before we go on holiday because I will only wear long sleeves and long skirts or trousers at times when my skin is unsightly. In fact, I cannot remember the last time I bought any summer clothes. I have a few dresses and tops which I can wear on holiday and for the weeks after we get back. Apart from that my choice of clothes is restricted to those which will conceal my patches of psoriasis. The choice is further limited by the fact that anything other than cotton is likely to irritate the skin.

I know that my psoriasis is relatively mild, and yet the effect it has on my self-confidence is enormous. The only time I feel really happy is in the summer when my psoriasis is cleared.

I have been too cowardly to take my children swimming in public pools because of my embarrassment at the state of my skin.

Since attending The Alternative Centre my condition has improved due to the treatment recommended, but also because I have been encouraged to take a more positive approach to my problem, and to believe that there is hope for the future. This contrasts sharply with the attitude encountered on a previous hospital visit which was basically: 'Your psoriasis is nowhere near as bad as some people's. Just be grateful and don't bother us again.'

### Dina Coverdale of Middlesex writes

Dear Sandra,

I am writing to thank you for the help and guidance I have received during my visits.

The counselling and constant support you have given me has taught me to look at myself, my lifestyle and those around me, my diet, my attitude towards myself, and my psoriasis in a completely positive way. Now, instead of feeling that I am different from anyone else and trying to cover up and keep apologising for my complaint, I accept it as a part of me, instead of living my life around it. It has now become a very small part of the rest of me. I am confident that I will cure myself of it, and am working towards that. Now that I have learnt what aggravates my skin (e.g. meat, dairy produce, chocolate, alcohol, etc.) I reduce these greatly, and feel so much better for it, too.

My whole attitude and way of life has changed thanks to you and Jane at The Alternative Centre. I am only sorry that I did not find you sooner.

Dina Coverdale is now working at The Alternative Centre. She is training to become a natural health consultant specialising in psoriasis with a view to opening a clinic in Sydney, Australia.

### From Mrs B of Wales

To all at The Alternative Centre

I would like to thank the staff at The Alternative Centre (especially Jane) for all their care and kindness in making me well.

I have been a sufferer of psoriasis for 22 years, during which time I have been in hospital six times, and have spent 2½ years on PUVA treatment for my psoriasis, which covered most of my body, arms, legs and scalp. After spending a few months with The Alternative Centre I am now much better than I have been for a long time.

### From Mrs J of Middlesex, England

Dear Toni,

I am just writing to thank you all so much for the help you have given my daughter. As you know, she had made many visits to the doctor and the hospital with her psoriasis before she came to you. Nothing seemed to help her, and she was in a very depressed state about everything. Within a few weeks of her treatment she was beginning to realize that there was help for her distressing condition.

She really thought that she would have to live with it, and try her best to get on with her life. Thanks to you she is almost clear of any patches, and feels so much better. It's almost a year now since I took her to see you, and I just wanted to let you know how Karla is now, and I just hope that many more people will turn to you for help.

Thank you once again.

### From Mr D of London

Dear Jane,

I am sorry I have not written sooner, but my psoriasis is greatly improved since I saw you in September. I am clear in many places and I have been swimming again. The diet has been hard but it's well worthwhile.

It was really good talking to you, and to hear a refreshing approach to psoriasis. Isn't it surprising that as recent as 1975 the *British Journal of Hospital Medicine* said 'Diet has no place in psoriasis'.

Kind regards

### From Miss L of Surrey

Dear Jane,

Just a few lines to let you know how I am progressing. I am up to three minutes each side on the UVB unit, and already my psoriasis has really improved.

My back, front and arms are now virtually free of any psoriasis. My legs are still quite bad, although much better than when I came to collect the unit. I've managed to cut down on tea and coffee and I don't have any problems with irritation like I used to.

In two weeks time I am due to see the skin specialist at the hospital. I do believe, though, by the time I see him my psoriasis will have gone. Once again Jane, thank you for all your help.

### From Mrs E of Sussex, England

Dear Centre

The purpose of this letter is to advise you that my son's skin has improved out of all recognition. His back is almost clear and his front is clearing slowly. I do hope that your 'formula' will continue to work, and that when the skin gets used to the preparations it does not break out all over again.

In any case, any remission is welcome. We have had our hopes raised in the past, and then the psoriasis comes back worse than before, and we hardly dare hope that after 12 years

we have found the answer.
Our many thanks for all your help.

## From Mrs W of Wales
Dear Sandra,
My daughter's skin is in perfect condition now. It's as if she never suffered from psoriasis, after eighteen years of always having it on her knees and elbows. It's nothing short of a miracle to see her skin soft and white without even a trace of dry skin.
Gratefully yours

## From Miss K of Cheshire, England
Dear Jane Waters,
My Corona unit arrived safely and I have been using it for about two weeks. Already I have obtained tremendous improvement, and each area of my psoriasis has 'shrunk' in size by at least half. I feel better than I have for years with much more confidence in myself – I have even bought a mini-skirt for summer; something which I have never been able to wear previously (and at 25 I can just get away with it!)
   With kindest regards to you all

## From Mrs C of Essex, England
Dear Sir or Madam,
I would just like to inform you that my treatment is going well after 20 years with psoriasis. It is very exciting to see it disappearing, and lots of patches have already completely gone. I am very grateful. Thank you.

## From Mrs D of South Wirral, England
Dear Sir/Madam,
I recently received from you the hair treatment, and for the first time in at least ten years I know what my real scalp looks like. In less than a week my scalp was clear and I am a much happier person. Because of this I can now go into a hairdresser and have my hair done, if I wish, instead of being too ashamed to go. I have a mobile hairdresser who has been very understanding in the past, and when I asked her to do my hair last weekend, she was so surprised because my scalp was clear.
   I just want to say a big thank you for a marvellous treatment.

**From Ms R of Surrey, England**

I have been a psoriasis sufferer since the age of ten, and have for the last fourteen years tried several treatments depending on the severity of my condition at the time. These treatments have included various tar-based products, steroid creams and the PUVA method. All have suppressed my psoriasis, none have been totally successful or pleasant.

The tar-based products are foul-smelling and messy to use, steroid creams are basically harmful used over a long period of time, and the PUVA method did not keep the condition at bay for any length of time at all. All, in their own, way have helped, but none have been as successful as a new Danish formula I have recently been using.

This formula is made from completely natural products, i.e. safe, is easy to apply and isn't foul-smelling – and, hallelujah, is working.

# Details of Conferences and Symposia on Psoriasis

Many of the drug-manufacturing companies financially contribute towards the running of Psoriasis Associations around the world which could explain the associations' reluctance to recommend alternative therapies. This is more applicable to the longer-established associations, and not more recently formed ones as I have encountered in Israel, Italy, Belgium and other countries. These are set up by well-meaning individuals supported by doctors or dermatologists whose main aim is recommending any therapy or treatment that will help the sufferers.

Doctors and dermatologists can only prescribe the treatments available to them, and mostly do so with caution. There is a tremendous amount of pressure associated with medical practice, as the public demand an instant cure for their problem. The patient wants to treat their condition as quickly as possible, and waits until they are sick before enlisting help.

However, many of the large drug companies are becoming more and more involved in natural medicine, buying out well-known existing companies and producing vitamins and other medicines. We are also seeing a change of attitude, more common in some countries than in others, in terms of preventative medicine amongst the public and doctors, with interest shown in stress-management therapies which can help to eliminate disease.

Recently, a medical delegation came to visit London from Russia, their purpose being to look at the field of alternative forms of medicine using in this country. Their main interest was in natural medicines which can be produced in their own country by scientists, for all nature of illness.

In Spain, in 1986, The 10th World Congress of Natural Medicines was attended by over 600 medical and alternative practitioners from all over the world. The participation of many eminent professors practising both orthodox and alternative medicine confirms that the two have been successfully combined for many years and the concept is not new.

I was invited to give a lecture, along with my colleague Jane Water, on the subjects of Living with Psoriasis and Psoriasis and Stress Management. Whilst attending the conference it soon became evident that many of these professional, extremely well-qualified people were genuinely interested in effective alternative ways to treat psoriasis.

Many of the doctors had been practising alternative medicine and natural therapies as a complementary contribution towards the health of their patients for years. It was seen as the 'normal' way to treat the sick.

Some of these therapies included: diet-therapy, electro-acupuncture; chiropractic; homoeopathy; meditation; holistic medicine; moratherapy; naturopathy; pulse diagnosis as in oriental medicine; laser therapy; Ayurveda; common herbs; magnetotherapy; massage; manipulation; ultrasonic therapy; Tibetan medicine; natural childbirth; hypnotherapy and many more.

One of the most interesting lectures, and there were many, was the Future of Natural and Traditional Medicines, given by V. N. Foster (U.K.) and J. M. Sanchez Perez (Mexico). Others included: African herbal medicine; New Clinical Methods by Jan De Vries (U.K.), one of our most renowned and respected experts, and The Relief of Pain by Han Chenggang (the People's Republic of China).

These regular events, taking place around the world, show the change of attitude towards a more holistic approach to treating disease which can successfully involve the medical and alternative field of medicine, and we are sure this trend will continue as we continue to demand no-risk treatments for our health.

The worldwide search for a cure for psoriasis is taking place every day by the top scientists in the world of dermatology. The answer has yet to be found. Meanwhile chemical and biological research is producing a wide range of new drugs and therapies, some of which have helped many severe sufferers.

To examine the progress of such research programmes, International Dermatology Conferences are held around the world. The first was held in Paris in 1889.

The First International Symposium on the Treatment of Psoriasis and Psoriatic-Arthritis was held in 1971. This conference was to examine findings, as well as treatments that had taken place during the previous ten years. Research carried out at Stanford, under the expert guidance of Professor E. M. Farber, world-famous for his work in dermatology, showed the multiple genetic factors and environmental stress that are necessary for the manifestation of psoriasis.

The conferences provide an opportunity for scientists from many countries to exchange ideas, allowing them to offer new information to those involved in treating psoriasis and the sufferers themselves. Their aim is to deal with psoriasis with compassion and scientific interest.

The Second International Symposium was held at Stanford University, California in 1976. For those of you interested in obtaining further information on the proceedings of this symposium on psoriasis, a book is available from Yorke Medical Books, in New York, entitled Psoriasis – Proceedings of the Second International Symposium.

Both the Third and Fourth Symposiums for Psoriasis and Psoriatic-Arthritis were held in Israel, in 1984 and 1989 respectively.

The conferences were sponsored by the International Psoriasis Treatment Centre at the Dead Sea, known for over ten years for successfully treating psoriasis sufferers, and the Department of Dermatology at Hadassah University Hospital, Jerusalem in collaboration with The Israel Dermatology Society.

I have selected a few abstracts from some of the lectures that I feel would be of general interest. Further information should be available from The Organising Committee, International Psoriasis Treatment Center, Israel.

*A Double-Blind, Randomised, Placebo-Controlled Trial of Fish Oil in Psoriasis*, S. S. Bleehen, S. B. Bittiner, I. Cartwright, W. F. G. Tucker, Departments of Dermatology and Haematology, Royal Hallamshire Hospital, Sheffield, U.K.

### Abstract

Eicosapentaenoic acid (EPA) is a 20-carbon polyunsaturated fatty acid that is structurally similar to arachidonic acid (AA). It is found almost exclusively in oils of marine origin and there have been several reports that it is of help in the treatment of patients with psoriasis. The patients in the two groups who completed 12 weeks of treatment were well matched for age, sex, disease duration and the type of topical treatments used. After 8 weeks there was a significant lessening of itching, erythema and scaling in the active treatment group, whereas there was no significant change in the control group given placebo capsules (olive oil).

*Dithranol for Psoriasis: A New Aqueous Gel Formulation* — M de la Brassine, J. P. Dechesne, A. Ghazi and L. Dellattre. Department of Dermatology, Laboratory of Galenical Pharmacy, University of Liège, Belgium.

### Abstract

Many disadvantages are linked with classical dithranol preparations: poor solubility of dithranol in water and aqueous vehicles, rapid oxydative degradation and bad cosmetic presentation. Adult patients suffering from localised psoriasis vulgaris were treated with new aqueous gel preparations containing an anthralin derivative. Patients were asked to apply 0.1% gel once a day for one week. Depending on the evolution of psoriasis lesions and on the tolerance in the surrounding skin, the concentration was increased or not during the next weeks. Clearing was obtained after just five weeks and no patient complained about the cosmetic tolerance.

*Fumaric Acid and Derivatives* — A New Modality of Treatment for Psoriasis by Dr Kremer, Pal Issak, Carmel Hospital, Haifa, Israel.

### Abstract

For several years the antipsoriatic effect of fumeric acid derivatives, particularly when taken internally, has been discussed. It has been presumed that fumarates which are present in the human cells as a endogenous, play a role in biochemical processes. Such treatment has been attributed with an antipsoriatic effect for the skin as well as joints. Controlled clinical trials of fumeric acid and derivatives in patients have been done and 50% to 60% success rate has been shown. Side effects appears in approximately 10% of patients but through dosage adjustment can be controlled.

Isolated cases of leukopenia and slight increase in kidney and liver function parameters were observed.

*Note:* Tests carried out in London in 1986 shown that the diet recommended with Fumeric Acid Therapy, at that time was responsible for improvement in the condition of psoriasis without taking to recommended daily dose of fumeric acid.

*Structuring the Self Care Process:* The Contribution of a Patient Association, by P. Labeeuw of Belgium Psoriasis Association, B 1700 Asse, Belgium.

## Abstract

A skin complaint is not to be reduced to a pure technical problem. It includes one's attitude towards the lesions and their effects on self-image. Self help groups offer to their members a pool of very practical and existential information which cannot be provided in the same experimental way by the professional. Both self-help and professional approaches are complementary and the issue of this brief communication is to show how they can be integrated.

*Pathogenesis and Treatment of Psoriasis:* Psychoneurophysiological Implications, by M. M. Polenghi, C. Gala, G. L. Manca and A. F. Finzi, 2nd Department of Dermatology, University of Milan, Italy.

## Abstract

Psoriasis is a skin disease whose pathogenesis often includes emotional-trauma factors. We have evaluated whether or not there is some connection between the autonomic nervous system response to a specific stress event and psoriasis. We have studied 100 psoriatic patients by semistructed interviews, psychometric tests (Paykel scale of stressful events, the MMPI test, the QTA test) and their psychophysiological profiles during a baseline period and during standard mental, emotional and physical stresses. Our results confirm the high incidence of stressful life events in the before the appearance of psoriasis.

*Alcohol Intake* — A Risk Factor for Psoriasis by T. Reunala, J. Lauharanta, J. Karvonen and K. Poikolainen, Departments of Dermatology, University Central Hospitals of Tampere, Helsinki and Oulu and National Public Health Inst., Helsinki, Finland.

### Abstract

An association between increased alcohol consumption and psoriasis has been suspected for years. We investigated the drinking habits of 51 male psoriatics (age 18-50 years). A detailed history of alcohol intake before and after the onset of psoriasis was taken for each patient and compared to that of 100 patients suffering from other dermatological disorders. Before contracting the disease, the average alcohol intake was 61 grams/day (100% alcohol) in psoriatics 48/51 and 37 grams/day in control patients. Almost all psoriatics (48/51) and controls (93/100) were drinkers and psoriatics reported being drunk on the average of 73 times and control patients 54 times per year. After contracting psoriasis, psoriatics increased slightly their alcohol intake, whereas the controls decreased their consumption.

*Immunesuppressive Effect of PUVA Therapy in Psoriatic Patients and Beneficial Effect of IL-2 in Vitro* by B. Shohat, M. David, A. Ingber, Cellular Immunology Unit and Department of Dermatology, Beilinson Medical Center, Petah Tikva, Israel.

### Abstract

PUVA therapy has a beneficial effect on psoriasis but may affect immune functions, possibly having carcinogenic potential. We undertook to test the effect of PUVA therapy on the cell mediated immunity of 50 psoriatic patients and the possibility of restoration of immune function.

During this enlightening conference we were introduced to a Professor Vladimozov, of the First Moscow Medical Institute in the USSR, who told us about the 3rd Symposium of Dermatology of the Socialist Countries on Psoriasis that was held in Moscow in 1987.

257 papers were submitted to the conference. Once again, I have selected an extract from some of the research papers that I feel will prove of the most interest to you.

*Management of Psoriasis;* Clinical Evidence of Justification by Yu Ya Ashmarin, Moscow.

### Abstract

The incidence of Psoriasis, which is a high as 2% of the world population, makes this disease a social problem. There is much irrefutable evidence that psoriasis is a disorder caused by a multitude factors, involving those pertaining to genetics and environment. The genesis of psoriasis is not yet clear. It must be confessed that genetic links are the only well-established fact of the etiology of the disease. The incidence of family psoriasis varies between 7% and 70% according to various authors. Predisposition to Psoriasis is associated with the genes of the main histocompatibility complex. An obvious relationship between the HLA system and some forms of psoriasis (pustular psoriasis and psoriatic arthropathy) has been noted.

*Psoriasis and Drugs,* N. Botev-Zlatkove, N. Tsankov, S. Tonev, A. Lazarova, L. Popova and M. Kostova, Sofia, Bulgaria.

### Abstract

447 psoriasis vulgaris patients were studied with the help of questionnaires, in order to find out the effect upon psoriasis of the drug therapy previously used on intercurrent disease. The authors report a considerable deterioration in the dermatological condition of the patients after treatments with beta-blockers, lithium, non steroidal analgesics, some antibiotics and vaccinations. Onset of psoriasis in 3 patients (0.67%) as well as exacerbation of the same disease in 15 patients — (3.35%) after treatment with tetracyline is described here — a fact which has not been discussed in medical literature until now. A control group of 100 patients with both psoriasis

and intercurrent diseases was also studied. 11% of the patients got deterioration of psoriasis during the course of influenza, tonsilitis, pharyngitis, sinusitis etc.

*Oral Retinoids and Thalassotherapy* (RE-SUN THERAPY) of Psoriasis by A. L. Dourmishev, N. B. Zlatkov, I. Ticholov, Sofia, Bulgaria.

## Abstract

36 psoriatics in 2 groups were treated with thalassotherapy on the Black Sea coast for 24 days. The patients from first group were given tigason (etretinate) orally 20mg/m$^2$ of skin surface. Free lipid acids in the blood serum of patients were examined prior to and after therapy. The second group of psoriatics were only treated with thalassotherapy and were a control group. Tigason combined with thalassotherapy — RE-SUN therapy in patients with psoriasis offers following advantages. A greater efficacy in patients unresponsive to thalasso-therapy alone. Improvement was obtained in reduced daily dosages of tigason and fewer side effects. A level of free lipid acids in the blood serum were unchanged after RE-SUN therapy.

*Spa Treatment of Psoriasis Patients in the Aric Climatic Zone* by A. M. Izmailov, S. S.Amaev, Ashkhabad, USSR.

## Abstract

The arid climate of the Turkmenia is a significant factor of psoriasis epidermiology and clinical development. Psoriasis is less among the aboriginal population than among newcomers. More cases are observed in the winter (32.5%), this number decreasing in the spring (20.7%) drastically reducing in the summer (13.2%) and autumn (15.7%); 17.9% of the patients show no seasonal preference. The clinical picture of psoriasis in the arid zone is relatively benign, with long remissions and rare complications.

*Psoriasis in the Structure of Skin Diseases in Children* by V. P. Kachanov, Leningrad, USSR.

## Abstract

The incidence of skin disease in children has been estimated the three ways. (1) analysis of medical records of the patients who applied for treatment (2) detecting the children with skin disease during selective examinations at preschool institutions and schools; (3) estimation of the number of children hospitalized at the clinic for skin diseases attached to the Leningrad Institute of Pediatrics.

*Treatment of Juvenile Pustular Psoriasis* by A. Kansky, P. Kmet-Vizintin, Z. Pavicic, Zagreb, Yugoslavia.

## Abstract

Generalised pustular psoriasis is rather rare in children under 10 years, according to Hubier less than 50 cases were published up to 1984. The treatment is difficult, according to our experience systemic application or corticosteroids should be avoided. 8 children with general pustular psoriasis of the Zambush type were admitted to the Children's Ward of our Department. Their age at the time of the treatment ranged from 3 to 11 years. The symptoms were similar in all patients: erythroderma studded with pustules, high fever, general malaise with signs of metabolic disturbances. All patients were treated previously to the pustular eruption with corticosteroids topically or orally.

*Drugs of Plant origin in the Combined Treatment of Psoriasis* by V. E. Korsun, N. A. Papiy, V. K. Zubritsky, Minsk, USSR.

## Abstract

A total of 151 patients with psoriasis were examined for the status of the gastrointestinal tract (uropepsin, amylase, enterokinase, peptidase levels), carbohydrate metabolism) proteinogram, bilirubin, lipoproteins, C-reactive protein), hormones (hydrocortisone, testosterone, dehydroepiandrosterone) immune status, (circulating immune complexes, T- and B- lymphocytes, immunoglobulin levels). A tincture of a collection of medicinal drugs of plant origin, approved by the Ministry of Health of the USSR was used for normalisation of gastric and hepatic functions in a dose of 100 ml twice a day after meals. Immunologic disorders were corrected by plant stimulants.

*Treatment of Psoriasis in a One-Day Hospital*, by O. A. Mashkov, G. YA Sharapova, V. A. Morgunov, V. V. Keremet, V. L. Moranelli, Moscow.

## Abstract

The number of reported cases of psoriasis is increasing as is the rate of the disability it causes. This necessitates search for new effective methods of its therapy. Hemoperfusion, used alone or together with the traditional methods of treatment, have been reported to result in clinical recovery or improvement in 68-78% of the patients, with remissions lasting for 6 months to 4 years. Hemoperfusion has been employed over a period of more than 5 years in the treatment of 876 patients with good clinical results and no complications or side effects. On the basis of this experience, the Moscow City Center of Hemoperfusion, with a one-day hospital, has been set up for patients with severe systemic dermatoses.

*Research Trends in Psoriasis* by F. Novtny, Prague, CSSR.

## Abstract

There are different research spheres and aims on psoriasis in several countries of the world. The bioregulatory questions predominate in pathogenic studies in the USA as well as the trend towards combined therapy. In the USSR there is a tendency to pathophysiology, biochemistry and practical treatment of psoriasis. In Czechoslovakia a tendency to genetics, psychotherapy and prevention of psoriasis relapses, in Poland and France the immunological studied are prevailing, in Hungary the biochemistry of cell membrane system, in western countries the ambulatory treatment in day care centres with phototherapy, anthralin ointment and cytostatics etc.

*Social and Economic Aspects of Psoriasis in Black Africa* by O. E. Obasi, Nigeria.

## Abstract

The disease of psoriasis is worldwide. Ethnic and racial factors have significant influence on its epidemiology. Therefore the epidemiology of psoriasis may not be fully appreciated without international co-operation and collaboration. The epidemiology of psoriasis in Black Africa is not fully understood. Available data are fragmentary and are contained in individual records of few dermatologists. Geographical and climatic factors have tremendous influence on its prevalence. Psoriasis is in general a mild disease with low morbidity in black Africans. The reason for this requires thorough investigation, the outcome of which could revolutionize the management of psoriasis. Despite the chronicity of the disease, patients in Nigeria (Africa) do not seek hospital treatment until they have exhausted all traditional methods, including witchcraft influence. Moreover, patients may suspect the disease to be leprosy, a dreaded disease that carries obvious social stigma.

In our experience certain factors such as high humidity and pregnancy appear to ameliorate the disease, while alcoholism worsens it. The traditional use of bathing fibres as sponge or the misguided use of 'antiseptic soaps' worsen the disease by producing a Koebner effect. The clinical features of psoriasis are the same as in caucasians but the colour of the disease seen on European skin is lost in the black skin. Psoriasis vulgaris with the typical morphological features may raise little or no diagnostic difficulties. But some aspects of the disease seen in black Africans in Nigeria, may present diagnostic dilemmas.

These extracts from the international field of psoriasis are just a glimpse of what takes place around the world each day. For those of you who would like more in-depth information, write to the recommended associations, whom I hope will be happy to forward information. Information from the conference in Russia may be obtainable from the All-Union Society of Dermatologists and Venereologists of the Ministry of Health of the USSR.

A very important contribution by Dr Terence J. Ryan, Consultant Dermatologists, John Radcliffe Hospital and Slade

Hospital, Oxford, England has come to my attention recently in the form of an article written, called *Handicap in Skin Disease* which I would like to finish this appendix with as it goes a long way to confirm a genuine concern, understanding and sympathy for the suffering associated with psoriasis, by many of the medical professionals.

### Abstract

1981 was the year of the International Concern for the Disabled, but in the account of its aims there was no mention of skin diseases. They are not seen as a cause for disablement. During the last few years in dealing with the allocation of finance by local authorities, parish charities and industries interested in making donations to the disabled, I have been perturbed at the fact that the book to which they turn has been the Directory for the Disabled which does not mention skin disease.

I spoke at a course for sexual problems of the disabled in 1981. This was the first time that such a course had included a talk on skin disease. I have noted that the handbooks for disablement settlement officers and advice given to local employment agencies, also similarly ignores skin diseases. More important, perhaps, the allocation of resources to regions in the United Kingdom has specifically left out skin diseases because it was recognised that their assessment is 'too complicated'.

There have been several articles in American journals drawing attention to the toll of skin diseases and, in particular, the cost to the individual, but all authors recognize the difficulties in quantifying the handicap. The scale of handicap in skin diseases is simply not known. Questions that may be asked include 'How far can someone walk if they have sore feet?'

How is manual dexterity interfered with when an electronics engineer develops psoriasis of the fingers? How is a commercial traveller affected by the fact that he leaves blood on the sheets and scales in the bathroom every time he visits the same hotel? How do we assess the handicap or the time taken to apply preparations to the skin to keep it reasonably respectable in appearance?'

If, as it is now well recognised, hand dermatitis is one of the worst handicaps with the respect to disablement then should we not be making more of this?

There are two aspects of skin disease which are not sufficiently known to the public. One is vulnerability. How much of a handicap is it if one is easily sunburned or develops chilblains in a cool room, or develops psoriasis when there is slight abrasion of the skin? The second and most important element that is missing in that of aversive handicap, or the problem of being unwelcome.

During the recent years of interest in mental handicaps the problem of being unwelcome has been better understood in regard of this disability. Perhaps only leprosy has an appropriate literature in the sphere of dermatology. It is a most difficult area to analyse, and one has to consider not only being actually unwelcome but imagining one is unwelcome.

In giving consideration to the degree of handicap, there are many questions that can be asked of the patient, and if one makes a habit of this one finds that some even with severe skin disease do not consider themselves handicapped at all. This also has important implications. What makes a patient handicapped? Is it the disease, or the society in which we live?

It is necessary to draw to the need for the measurement of handicap in order to introduce our subject more convincingly to those who provide the resources for training of social workers and nurses, and even to give consideration to the manner in which some treatments are themselves the source of handicap. Words such as access, vulnerability and mobility are as important in dermatology as they are in other areas of disablement.

# Further reading

*Complete Nutrition*, Michael Sharon (Prion/Multi-Media Books)
*Super Foods*, Michael Van Straten and Barbara Griggs (Dorling Kindersley)
*Fit for Life*, Harvey and Marilyn Diamond (Bantam)
*Food Combining for Health*, Doris Grant and Jean Joice (Thorsons)
*Food Combining for Vegetarians*, Jackie Le Tissier (Thorsons)
*Living with Psoriasis*, Sandra Gibbons (Alternative Centre Publications)
*Love is Never Enough*, Aaron T. Beck (Penguin)
*Love, Medicine and Miracles* and *Peace, Love and Miracles*, Bernie S. Seigel (Rider)
*Vaccination and Immunisation*, Leon Chaitow (C. W. Daniel)
*Power of Unconditional Love*, Ken Keyes Jnr (Love Line Books, USA)
*The Singing Detective*, Dennis Potter (Faber & Faber)
*Autogenic Training* (Chapter 3), Kai Kermani (Thorsons)
*Iridology*, Adam Jackson (Optima)
*Dance of Anger*, Harriet Goldhor Lerner (Thorsons)
*Proceedings of the Second International Symposium of Psoriasis* (Faber & Cox, Yorke Medical Books, 666 Fifth Avenue, New York)

## Books for teenagers
*It's More Than Sex:* A survival guide to the teenage years, Suzie Hayman (Wildwood House)
*The New Our Bodies, Ourselves:* A health book by and for women, Angela Phillips and Jill Rakusen (Penguin)
*The Teenage Body Book:* Honest, no-nonsense answers to the hundreds of questions you have always wanted to ask, Kathy McCoy & Dr Charles Wibbelsman (Piatkus)

In addition to letters from psoriasis sufferers, The Alternative Centre receives requests daily from medical practitioners all over the world, wanting further information about psoriasis treatment and the services we offer. We pride ourselves on helping to bridge the gap between conventional and alternative practice to bring relief to our patients. The following letter regarding *Living with Psoriasis* is one of my favourites:

> Dear Sirs,
> I have shown the book Living with Psoriasis to a large number of patients and no doubt you will see from your records that a considerable number have sent for a copy of this useful contribution, by Sandra Gibbons. However, one of my patients has walked off with my copy so I do wonder whether it would be at all possible for you to send another copy. If you do I presume it would be best if I chained it to the desk this time. With very many thanks.
>
> Mr J, Consultant Dermatologist
> Vale of Leven District General Hospital  February 1987

For more information on the holistic approach to psoriasis contact:

The Alternative Centre
The White House
Roxby Place
Fulham
LONDON SW6 1RS

Phone: 071-381 2298

# Index